Cognitive Behavioral Therapy

Editors

RIANNE A. DE KLEINE
JASPER A.J. SMITS
STEFAN G. HOFMANN

PSYCHIATRIC CLINICS
OF NORTH AMERICA

www.psych.theclinics.com

Consulting Editor
HARSH K. TRIVEDI

June 2024 • Volume 47 • Number 2

ELSEVIER

1600 John F. Kennedy Boulevard • Suite 1800 • Philadelphia, Pennsylvania, 19103-2899

http://www.theclinics.com

PSYCHIATRIC CLINICS OF NORTH AMERICA Volume 47, Number 2
June 2024 ISSN 0193-953X, ISBN-13: 978-0-443-24682-1

Editor: Megan Ashdown
Developmental Editor: Varun Gopal

Psychiatric Clinics of North America (ISSN 0193-953X) is published quarterly by Elsevier Inc., 360 Park Avenue South, New York, NY 10010-1710. Months of issue are March, June, September, and December. Business and Editorial Offices: 1600 John F. Kennedy Blvd., Suite 1800, Philadelphia, PA 19103-2899. Periodicals postage paid at New York, NY and additional mailing offices. Subscription prices are $362.00 per year (US individuals), $100.00 per year (US students/residents), $422.00 per year (Canadian individuals), $535.00 per year (international individuals), and $220.00 per year (international students/residents), $100.00 per year (Canadian & students/residents). For institutional access pricing please contact Customer Service via the contact information below. Foreign air speed delivery is included in all *Clinics'* subscription prices. All prices are subject to change without notice. **POSTMASTER:** Send address changes to *Psychiatric Clinics of North America*, Elsevier Health Sciences Division, Subscription Customer Service, 3251 Riverport Lane, Maryland Heights, MO 63043. **Customer Service: 1-800-654-2452 (US). From outside the United States, call 1-314-447-8871. Fax: 1-314-447-8029. E-mail: journalscustomerservice-usa@elsevier.com (for print support) and journalsonlinesupport-usa@elsevier.com (for online support).**

Reprints. For copies of 100 or more, of articles in this publication, please contact the Commercial Reprints Department, Elsevier Inc., 360 Park Avenue South, New York, New York 10010-1710. Tel.: 212-633-3874, Fax: 212-633-3820, E-mail: reprints@elsevier.com.

Psychiatric Clinics of North America is covered in *MEDLINE/PubMed (Index Medicus), Current Contents/Social and Behavioral Sciences, Social Science Citation Index, Embase/Excerpta Medica,* and PsycINFO.

Contributors

CONSULTING EDITOR

HARSH K. TRIVEDI, MD, MBA
President and Chief Executive Officer, Sheppard Pratt Health System, Baltimore, Maryland, USA

EDITORS

RIANNE A. DE KLEINE, PhD
Assistant Professor, Clinical Psychology, Leiden University, Leiden, Netherlands

JASPER A.J. SMITS, PhD
Professor, Department of Psychology, The University of Texas at Austin, Austin, Texas, USA

STEFAN G. HOFMANN, PhD
Alexander von Humboldt Professor, LOEWE Spitzenprofessur für Translationale Klinische Psychologie, Philipps-University of Marburg, Marburg, Germany

AUTHORS

JONATHAN S. ABRAMOWITZ, PhD
Professor, Department of Psychology, The University of North Carolina at Chapel Hill, Chapel Hill, North Carolina, USA

REBECCA A. ANDERSON, PhD
Senior Lecturer, School of Population Health and enAble Institute, Curtin University, Bentley, Western Australia, Australia

JOANNA J. ARCH, PhD
Professor, Department of Psychology and Neuroscience, University of Colorado Boulder, Boulder, Colorado, USA

MELISSA BLACK, PhD
Clinical Research Lead, School of Psychology, UNSW Sydney, Sydney, New South Wales, Australia; Black Dog Institute, Randwick, New South Wales, Australia

ANNAMARIE DEMARCO, BS
Senior Research Associate, Department of Psychiatry and Behavioral Sciences, Center for Psychedelic Research and Therapy, The University of Texas at Austin Dell Medical School, Austin, Texas, USA

LAURA J. DIXON, PhD
Associate Professor, Department of Psychology, University of Mississippi, Mississippi, USA

LAUREN ENTEN, BSA
Senior Research Coordinator, Department of Psychiatry and Behavioral Sciences, Center for Psychedelic Research and Therapy, The University of Texas at Austin Dell Medical School, Austin, Texas, USA

GREGORY A. FONZO, PhD
Assistant Professor, Department of Psychiatry and Behavioral Sciences, Center for Psychedelic Research and Therapy, The University of Texas at Austin Dell Medical School, Austin, Texas, USA

BRONWYN M. GRAHAM, PhD
Professor, School of Psychology, UNSW Sydney, Sydney, New South Wales, Australia

SAIDA HESHMATI, PhD
Assistant Professor, Department of Psychology, Claremont Graduate University, Claremont, California, USA

STEFAN G. HOFMANN, PhD
Alexander von Humboldt Professor, LOEWE Spitzenprofessur für Translationale Klinische Psychologie, Philipps-University of Marburg, Marburg, Germany

JÜRGEN HOYER, PhD
Professor, Technische Universitaet Dresden, Dresden, Germany

JONATHAN D. HUPPERT, PhD
Professor, Department of Psychology, The Hebrew University of Jerusalem, Mt Scopus, Jerusalem, Israel

NUSRAT HUSAIN, MD
Professor, Department of Psychiatry, University of Manchester, Manchester, England

JOLENE JACQUART, PhD
Clinical Assistant Professor, Department of Psychology, The University of Arizona, Tucson, Arizona, USA

DAVID JOHNSON, BS
Department of Psychological and Brain Sciences, Texas A&M University, College Station, Texas, USA

NIKOLAOS KAZANTZIS, PhD, FAPS, BICBT-CC
Professor of Clinical Psychology and Principal Researcher, Cognitive Behavior Therapy Research Unit, Melbourne, Victoria, Australia; Beck Institute for Cognitive Behavior Therapy, Philadelphia, Pennsylvania, USA

RACHEL KLINE, BA
Senior Research Associate, Department of Psychiatry and Behavioral Sciences, Center for Psychedelic Research and Therapy, The University of Texas at Austin Dell Medical School, Austin, Texas, USA

KELLY A. KNOWLES, PhD
Postdoctoral Fellow, The Institute of Living, Hartford Hospital, Hartford, Connecticut, USA

JENNIFER KRAFFT, PhD
Assistant Professor, Department of Psychology, Mississippi State University, Mississippi State, Mississippi, USA

MADELINE L. KUSHNER, BA
Department of Psychology, University of Kentucky, Lexington, Kentucky, USA

LEWIS LEONE, MS
Practicum Student Therapist, Department of Psychology, The University of Texas at Austin, Austin, Texas, USA

MICHAEL E. LEVIN, PhD
Professor, Department of Psychology, Utah State University, Logan, Utah, USA

KAYLA A. LORD, PhD
Psychologist, The Institute of Living, Hartford Hospital, Hartford, Connecticut, USA

ELIZABETH MASON, PhD
Professor, Clinical Research Unit for Anxiety and Depression, St Vincent's Health Network, Darlinghurst, New South Wales, Australia

PETER M. McEVOY, PhD
Professor, Centre for Clinical Interventions, Perth, Western Australia, Australia

DEAN McKAY, PhD
Professor, Department of Psychology, Fordham University, Bronx, New York, USA

BRYAN McSPADDEN, BA
Research Coordinator, Department of Psychology, The University of Texas at Austin, Austin, Texas, USA

FAROOQ NAEEM, PhD
Professor, Department of Psychiatry, University of Toronto, Toronto, Ontario, Canada

JILL M. NEWBY, PhD
Associate Professor, School of Psychology, Lecturer, UNSW Sydney, Black Dog Institute, Randwick, New South Wales, Australia

MICHAEL W. OTTO, PhD
Professor, Department of Psychological and Brain Sciences, Boston University, Boston, Massachusetts, USA

SANTIAGO PAPINI, PhD
Assistant Professor, Department of Psychology, University of Hawai'i at Mānoa, Honolulu, Hawai, USA

PETER PHIRI, PhD
Visiting Academic, Psychology Department, University of Southampton, Southampton, England

ANDRE PITTIG, PhD
Professor, Translational Psychotherapy, Institute of Psychology, University of Goettingen, Göttingen, Germany

WINFRIED RIEF, PhD
Professor, Department of Psychology, University of Marburg, Marburg, Germany

DAVID ROSENFIELD, PhD
Professor, Department of Psychology, Southern Methodist University, Dallas, Texas, USA

SHANNON SAUER-ZAVALA, PhD
Associate Professor, Department of Psychology, University of Kentucky, Lexington, Kentucky, USA

GUDMUNDUR SKARPHEDINSSON, PhD
Professor, Faculty of Psychology, University of Iceland, Reykjavik, Iceland

ORRI SMÁRASON, PhD
Clinical Psychologist and Researcher, Department of Child and Adolescent Psychiatry, Landspitali – The National University Hospital of Iceland, Reykjavik, Iceland

JASPER A.J. SMITS, PhD
Professor, Department of Psychology, The University of Texas at Austin, Austin, Texas, USA

MATTHEW W. SOUTHWARD, PhD
Assistant Professor, Department of Psychology, University of Kentucky, Lexington, Kentucky, USA

ERIC A. STORCH, PhD
Professor, Menninger Department of Psychiatry and Behavioral Sciences, Baylor College of Medicine, Houston, Texas, USA

DOUGLAS R. TERRILL, MS
Research Assistant, Department of Psychology, University of Kentucky, Lexington, Kentucky, USA

KIARA R. TIMPANO, PhD
Assistant Professor, Department of Psychology, The University of Miami, Coral Gables, Florida, USA

DAVID F. TOLIN, PhD
Director, Anxiety Disorders Center, The Institute of Living, Hartford Hospital, Hartford, Connecticut, USA; Yale University School of Medicine, New Haven, Connecticut, USA

MICHAEL P. TWOHIG, PhD
Professor, Department of Psychology, Utah State University, Logan, Utah, USA

EMILY UPTON, M. Psych (Clinical)
Clinical Psychologist, Black Dog Institute, Randwick, New South Wales, Australia

ANDRE WANNEMÜLLER, PhD
Researcher, Mental Health Research and Treatment Center, Ruhr University Bochum, Bochum, Germany

MARLON WESTHOFF, MSc
Research Fellow, Department of Psychology, Philipps-University of Marburg, Translational Clinical Psychology Group, Marburg, Germany

Contents

> In this article, the authors critically evaluate contemporary models of psychopathology and therapies, underscoring the limitations of traditional symptom-based classification approaches in mental health. The authors introduce a paradigm shift in the field, toward a process-oriented and dynamic systems approach to psychotherapy that offers deeper insights into the complex interplay of symptoms and individual experiences in psychopathology. These approaches offer a more personalized and effective understanding and treatment of mental health issues, moving beyond static and 1-dimensional views. The authors discuss the implications for clinical practice, emphasizing improved assessment, diagnosis, and tailored treatment strategies.

> Treatment engagement, crucial in cognitive behavioral therapy (CBT) outcomes, centers on consistent implementation of between-session homework. This article explores clinical features affecting engagement, including challenges related to psychosocial stressors and negative core beliefs. Empirical evidence supports the positive causal and correlational relationship between homework and symptom reduction. Recent studies highlight the role of patient beliefs and suggest a collaborative approach in homework design. The CBT account of treatment engagement emphasizes clinician behavior, patient beliefs, and task specificity. The comprehensive model of homework in CBT involves careful planning, collaborative review, and addressing patient-specific challenges, providing valuable clinical insights.

> Anxiety and depression are prevalent and impairing psychiatric problems for children and adolescents. In this review, the authors summarize information about their prevalence and impact, the most common assessment methods, the main components of cognitive behavioral therapy (CBT), and research on the effectiveness of CBT for these disorders. Future directions, including improving access to CBT through technology-based approaches and increasing personalization of treatment, are discussed.

Cultural values, traditions, and norms influence the practice of psychotherapy. It is now widely accepted that modern evidence-based therapies such
as CBT need to be culturally adapted for them to be successfully applied to
clients from a non-Western background. There are multiple factors to support cultural adaptations, such as evidence from research and an increase in
cultural awareness and globalization. A number of meta-analyses supporting culturally adapted interventions have been published across the globe. A
review of these meta-analyses reported that culturally adapted interventions
have moderate to high effect sizes in favor of culturally adapted psychological interventions. We provide a brief background on cultural differences and
suggest ways to address these differences. We also discuss the current
state of science in this area. We also provide a brief description of factors
that are generally accepted as important components of culturally adapted
interventions. We discuss the Southampton Adaptation Framework widely
used to Culturally adapt CBT (SAF-CaCBT). This framework has been
used in South Asia, the Middle East, China, England, Africa, and Canada.
More than 20 studies have used the framework to adapt CBT culturally.
The framework has evolved based on lessons learned from research and
consists of 3 major areas of concern: awareness of culture and religion, assessment and engagement, and adjustments in therapy. Each area has 8
subareas to consider when culturally adapting CBT. Finally, we discuss
the limitations and barriers in this area and recommendations for future
work. There is a need to develop universal guidelines on cultural adaptation
as well as areas of adaptation, more research with better methodology and
the use of active comparators in the assessment of culturally adapted interventions. There is also a need to further strengthen the evidence base by robust meta analyses.

Cognitive behavior therapies (CBTs) are the gold standard treatment for
many psychiatric conditions. However, relatively little is known about
how CBTs work. By characterizing these mechanisms, researchers can
ensure CBTs retain their potency across diagnoses and delivery contexts.
We review 3 classes of putative mechanisms: CBT-specific skills (eg, cognitive restructuring, behavioral activation), transtheoretical mechanisms
(eg, therapeutic alliance, treatment expectancies, self-efficacy beliefs),
and psychopathological mechanisms (aversive reactivity, positive affect,
attachment style). We point to future research within each class and emphasize the need for more intensive longitudinal designs to capture how
each class of mechanisms interacts with the others to improve outcomes.

We review the literature on various strategies to augment cognitive-behavioral therapy (CBT). Although traditional pharmacotherapy has only

a small additive effect, research demonstrates that it is possible to select interventions that potentiate known mechanisms of CBT. D-cycloserine appears to potentiate activity at the N-methyl D-ethyl aspartate receptor and thereby facilitates fear extinction. Exercise may increase neural plasticity and thereby increase the efficacy of CBT for depression and anxiety. Noninvasive brain stimulation is thought to target the specific cortical regions needed for CBT response, but results have been mixed. Several other compounds appear promising but await controlled research before their efficacy as an augmentation strategy can be determined.

> Administration of psychedelics for mental health treatment, typically referred to as "psychedelic-assisted therapy," is a broad term with a very heterogeneous implementation. Despite increasing interest in the clinical application of psychedelic compounds for psychiatric disorders, there is no consensus on how to best integrate the psychedelic experience with evidence-based psychotherapeutic treatment. This systematic review provides a timely appraisal of existing approaches to combining psychotherapy with psychedelics and provides clear recommendations to best develop, optimize, and integrate evidence-based psychotherapy with psychedelic administration for straightforward scientific inference and maximal therapeutic benefit.

> Technology-delivered cognitive behavioral therapy (CBT) has enabled more people to access effective, affordable mental health care. This study provides an overview of the most common types of technology-delivered CBT, including Internet-delivered, smartphone app, and telehealth CBT, as well as their evidence for the treatment of a range of mental health conditions. We discuss gaps in the existing evidence and future directions in the field for the use of technology CBT interventions.

> This review summarized recent systematic reviews and meta-analyses on randomized controlled trials evaluating acceptance and commitment therapy (ACT). Although the strength of evidence varies, overall there is plausible evidence for the efficacy of ACT for a wide range of areas including depression, anxiety disorders, obsessive-compulsive and related disorders, psychosis, substance use disorders, chronic pain, coping with chronic health conditions, obesity, stigma, and stress and burnout. ACT is also efficacious when delivered in digital self-help formats. Reviews of mediation research indicate ACT works through increasing psychological flexibility.

Jasper A.J. Smits, Jonathan S. Abramowitz, Joanna J. Arch, Santiago Papini,
Rebecca A. Anderson, Laura J. Dixon, Bronwyn M. Graham, Stefan G. Hofmann,
Jürgen Hoyer, Jonathan D. Huppert, Jolene Jacquart, David Johnson,
Peter M. McEvoy, Dean McKay, Jill Newby, Michael W. Otto, Andre Pittig,
Winfried Rief, David Rosenfield, Kiara R. Timpano, and Andre Wannemüller

The Exposure Therapy Consortium (ETC) was established to advance the science and practice of exposure therapy. To encourage participation from researchers and clinicians, this article describes the organizational structure and activities of the ETC. Initial research working group experiences and a proof-of-principle study underscore the potential of team science and larger-scale collaborative research in this area. Clinical working groups have begun to identify opportunities to enhance access to helpful resources for implementing exposure therapy effectively. This article discusses directions for expanding the consortium's activities and its impact on a global scale.

PSYCHIATRIC CLINICS OF NORTH AMERICA

FORTHCOMING ISSUES

September 2024
Crisis Services
Margie Balfour and Matthew Goldman, *Editors*

December 2024
Anxiety Disorders
Jordan Stiede and Eric Storch, *Editors*

March 2025
Psychiatric Genomics: Recent Advances and Clinical Implications
James J. Crowley, *Editor*

RECENT ISSUES

March 2024
Sleep Disorders in Children and Adolescents
Jessica Lunsford-Avery and Argelinda Baroni, *Editors*

December 2023
Adolescent Cannabis Use
Paula Riggs, Jesse D. Hinckley and J. Megan Ross, *Editors*

September 2023
Women's Mental Health
Susan G. Kornstein and Anita H. Clayton, *Editors*

SERIES OF RELATED INTEREST

Child and Adolescent Psychiatric Clinics of North America
https://www.childpsych.theclinics.com/

Neurologic Clinics
https://www.neurologic.theclinics.com/

Advances in Psychiatry and Behavioral Health
https://www.advancesinpsychiatryandbehavioralhealth.com/

THE CLINICS ARE AVAILABLE ONLINE!
Access your subscription at:
www.theclinics.com

PSYCHIATRIC CLINICS OF
NORTH AMERICA

SERIES OF RELATED INTEREST

Preface

Advancements in Cognitive Behavioral Therapy

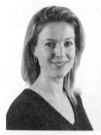 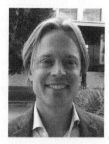 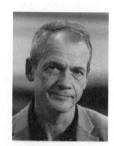

Rianne A. de Kleine, PhD   Jasper A.J. Smits, PhD   Stefan G. Hofmann, PhD

Editors

Cognitive behavioral therapy (CBT) represents a collection of treatment approaches designed to address and overcome mental health problems. CBT stands out as the most extensively studied psychological treatment for depression[1] and anxiety disorders,[2,3] and it is recommended in most treatment guidelines worldwide. Beyond these prevalent mental health issues, CBT programs have been tailored to address nearly all psychiatric symptoms.[4] Despite its demonstrated effectiveness, there remains room for improvement, as not all patients respond positively to treatment. In response to this challenge, the field has explored avenues for enhancement in recent years.

The question of whether a diagnostic approach to mental health problems, with latent disease entities treated with specific therapy protocols, is still viable for clinical practice and research is an important one.[5] Indeed, the field is transitioning toward a transdiagnostic approach in which specific symptoms and their interrelations are central. This shift coincides with a heightened interest in understanding the mechanisms underlying CBT's effects. The examination of change mechanisms necessitates greater precision in the application of CBT procedures and the approach to evaluating therapeutic change. This is especially relevant in the context of (pharmacologic) augmentation studies that aim to evaluate the efficacy of strategies that target CBT mechanisms, such as extinction learning or extinction retention.

Another noteworthy development is the increasing impact of digital innovations. First, this transformation influences the accessibility and delivery of CBT interventions. Those suffering from psychological problems can now easily access CBT-based apps and digital interventions, a trend notably accelerated by the response to the COVID-19 pandemic. Second, digital innovations have influenced CBT research, with the availability of software allowing for fine-grained testing of CBT effects on an individual patient level (eg, through ecological moment assessment). Advances in statistical methods, coupled with improved accessibility through open-source software

Psychiatr Clin N Am 47 (2024) xiii–xv

https://doi.org/10.1016/j.psc.2024.03.001

0193-953X/24/© 2024 Elsevier Inc. All rights reserved.

packages and data-sharing initiatives, have shaped the evaluation of treatment effects and holds promise in providing a more meticulous understanding of who, under what circumstances, is likely to respond positively to CBT treatment.

Focused on these developments, this issue starts by reviewing novel developments in studying mechanisms in CBT (by Saida Heshmati, and colleagues). This is followed by articles on strategies for enhancing treatment engagement in CBT (by Nikolaos Kazantzis and colleagues), CBT for anxiety and depression in children and adolescents (by Orri Smárason, and colleagues), and cultural adaptations of CBT (by Farooq Naeem, and colleagues). Recent developments are further discussed in articles focusing on transdiagnostic mechanisms in CBT (by Matthew W. Southward, and colleagues), pharmacologic augmentation (by David F. Tolin, and colleagues), psychedelics and CBT (by Lewis Leone, and colleagues), technology-based CBT (by Jill M. Newby, and colleagues), and acceptance and commitment therapy (by Michael E. Levin, and colleagues). Last, the final article (in this issue by Jasper Smits and colleagues) discusses how closer collaboration and rigor in research procedures could move the CBT field forward. We think this issue offers an indicative overview of the current status and future directions of CBT.

Rianne A. de Kleine, PhD
Clinical Psychology
Leiden University
Leiden, Netherlands

Jasper A.J. Smits, PhD
Department of Psychology
The University of Texas at Austin
Austin, TX, USA

Stefan G. Hofmann, PhD
LOEWE Spitzenprofessur für
Translationale Klinische Psychologie
Philipps–Universität Marburg
Marburg, Germany

E-mail addresses:
r.a.de.kleine@fsw.leidenuniv.nl (R.A. de Kleine)
smits@utexas.edu (J.A.J. Smits)
stefan.g.hofmann@gmail.com (S.G. Hofmann)

REFERENCES

1. Cuijpers P, Miguel C, Harrer M, et al. Cognitive behavior therapy vs. control conditions, other psychotherapies, pharmacotherapies and combined treatment for depression: a comprehensive meta-analysis including 409 trials with 52,702 patients. World Psychiatry 2023;22(1):105–15. https://doi.org/10.1002/wps.21069.

2. Carpenter JK, Andrews LA, Witcraft SM, et al. Cognitive behavioral therapy for anxiety and related disorders: a meta-analysis of randomized placebo-controlled trials. Depress Anxiety 2018;35(6):502–14. https://doi.org/10.1002/da.22728.

3. van Dis EAM, van Veen SC, Hagenaars MA, et al. Long-term outcomes of cognitive behavioral therapy for anxiety-related disorders: a systematic review and meta-analysis. JAMA Psychiatry 2020;77(3):265–73. https://doi.org/10.1001/jamapsychiatry.2019.3986.

4. Hofmann SG, Asnaani A, Vonk IJJ, et al. The efficacy of cognitive behavioral ther-apy: a review of meta-analyses. Cognit Ther Res 2012;36(5):427–40. https://doi.org/10.1007/s10608-012-9476-1.
5. Hofmann SG, Hayes SC. The future of intervention science: process-based therapy. Clin Psychol Sci 2019;7(1):37–50. https://doi.org/10.1177/2167702618772296.

Novel Approaches Toward Studying Change

Implications for Understanding and Treating Psychopathology

Saida Heshmati, PhD[a],*, Marlon Westhoff, MSc[b],
Stefan G. Hofmann, PhD[b]

KEYWORDS

- Psychopathology • Psychotherapy • Evidence-based therapy
- Processes of change • Idiography • Ecological momentary assessment
- Dynamic network analysis

KEY POINTS

- Traditional models of psychopathology, based on symptom-based classifications, are limited in addressing the dynamic and individualized nature of mental health.
- This article emphasizes the need for idiographic and process-oriented approaches, moving away from static models to dynamic and personalized systems of psychopathology and health.
- The article explores alternative methodologies, such as process-based therapy, dynamic network modeling, and control theory, which offer deeper insights into the interplay of symptoms and underlying mechanisms in mental health disorders.

Easing human suffering is a formidable endeavor, necessitating robust conceptual frameworks to distill complexity into manageable issues. The way mental health problems are conceptualized and classified fundamentally influences the clinician's views and therapeutic approach to these problems. Nosology, the taxonomy of mental diseases, relies on methodological tools enabling the extraction of universal insights from diverse individual experiences. The primary objective of clarifying a person's psychopathology is to facilitate the provision of the most effective treatment tailored to their unique needs. However, contemporary approaches to understanding and treating psychopathology and mental health have encountered significant challenges and

[a] Department of Psychology, Claremont Graduate University, 150 E. 10th Street, Claremont, CA 91711, USA; [b] Department of Psychology, Philipps-University of Marburg, Translational Clinical Psychology Group, Schulstraße 12, Marburg D-35032, Germany
* Corresponding author.
E-mail address: saida.heshmati@cgu.edu

Psychiatr Clin N Am 47 (2024) 287–300
https://doi.org/10.1016/j.psc.2024.02.001
0193-953X/24/© 2024 Elsevier Inc. All rights reserved.

psych.theclinics.com

limitations. In this article, we critically examine the current paradigms in psychopathology and mental health treatment, and propose an alternative approach that seeks to address these shortcomings. Our goal is to pave the way for a more effective, empathetic, and nuanced approach to mental health care, ultimately enhancing our ability to alleviate human suffering.

CONTEMPORARY MODELS OF PSYCHOPATHOLOGY AND THERAPIES
The Latent Disease Model of Psychiatry

Psychiatry and behavioral sciences both share the aim of alleviating human suffering but differ in the initial foundational paradigms and associated methodologies. Psychiatry has been classifying psychopathology under the assumption that an individual's problems are symptoms of 1 or more latent disease entities. Psychopathology in psychiatric classification systems is described as "a syndrome marked by clinically significant disruption in an individual's cognition, emotion regulation, or behavior, indicating a dysfunction in the psychological, biological, or developmental processes that underlie mental functioning."[1 (p20)] With this definition, the Diagnostic and Statistical Manual of Mental Disorders (DSM) adopted a disease model to equate mental diseases as "dysfunctions." It further assumes the existence of "processes that underlie mental functioning," pointing to latent disease etiologies. The dysfunctional latent processes are manifested in the form of symptoms that are then grouped into syndromes to define the specific psychopathology.

The initial editions of the DSM were heavily influenced by psychoanalytic theory, positing that psychopathology stemmed from profound inner conflicts. Subsequent editions, reflecting a shift in perspective, were shaped by biologically oriented psychiatrists. These professionals explored the role of genetics, neuropeptides, brain circuitries, and other biological markers in determining the root causes of mental diseases.

Despite extensive research over many years, investigations into the biological underpinnings of psychopathology have not yielded significant results, largely due to a range of clinical and theoretic challenges. For instance, 1 key issue is the necessity to adhere to the axiom of local independence for validating the hypothesis that a latent variable is responsible for the co-occurrence of symptoms. The observed covariance among symptoms should only be attributable to the underlying disorder, and not to direct causal relationships between the symptoms themselves. In other words, when the presence of the disorder is accounted for, the correlations among symptoms should no longer be significant.

This condition is clearly demonstrated in certain physical health conditions. For example, in lung cancer, symptoms such as coughing, chest pain, breathlessness, and chest discomfort are interconnected; however, this correlation is primarily due to the presence of a tumor. When the tumor is considered, these symptoms no longer show a direct correlation with each other. Similarly, in Down syndrome, symptoms like intellectual deficiency, a crease across the palm, short stature, and a protruding tongue co-occur because they share a common cause, namely 3 copies of chromosome 21. In this case, there are no direct causal relations between individual symptoms, such as between short stature and a protruding tongue.

This clarity of causal relationships in physical conditions contrasts with the complexities and ambiguities often found in mental health disorders, where such straightforward causal links between symptoms and underlying biological factors are less evident. For example, in depression, a person who engages in excessive rumination may frequently suffer from insomnia. This lack of sleep, in turn, can lead to fatigue, which negatively impacts concentration and further lowers mood the next day. These interconnected symptoms demonstrate a chain of cause and effect within the syndrome of depression, complicating the application of both latent categorical and latent dimensional models of psychopathology. Such models typically rely on the assumption that symptom covariance is primarily due to a common underlying factor, an assumption that does not hold up well in the face of these evident causal relationships among symptoms in psychiatric conditions. This complexity highlights the challenges in understanding and modeling mental health disorders, where symptoms are often interdependent in a way that defies simple categorization or dimensional analysis.

Understanding Therapeutic Change

The exploration of therapeutic change in clinical science has long been a subject of intense study and debate. Central to this exploration is the understanding of how and why therapy works, which involves dissecting the intricate processes and mechanisms at play. This quest for understanding has led to the development of various models and theories, among which the concepts of mediators and moderators have become particularly influential.

Baron and Kenny's[2] article, published in 1986, introduced these terms to the field of psychology. Using simple and elegant methods with linear regressions to study mediation of change gained immense popularity. Their straightforward "causal steps" approach to study mediation and moderation was summarized in their 1986 article published in the *Journal of Social and Personality Psychology*, which became 1 of the top 100 most cited articles of all time in the entire field of science,[3] surpassing numerous Nobel prize–winning papers in chemistry and biology in terms of total citations. Their approach has brought several advantages to the field of research.

However, despite its widespread acceptance and influence, the Baron and Kenny model has its limitations, especially in clarifying the mechanisms and processes of psychotherapy. As noted elsewhere,[4] the authors believe that the linear mediation approach, with its assumptions of linearity and unidirectionality, falls short in capturing the intricate nature of treatment processes. It is further assumed that there are only some variables responsible for change processes. The model's reliance on paucivariate approaches (containing only a few variables) is seen as inadequate for a comprehensive examination of treatment processes. In contrast, methods that can examine the connection between multiple variables, including 2-way relationships that change in a non-linear and dynamic manner due to treatment, are required. This shift in perspective calls for a more nuanced and multifaceted approach to understanding therapeutic change.

The Role of the Individual

To effectively comprehend and treat psychopathology, it is crucial to focus on the individual, as each person's experience with a disorder is unique. Traditional research methods often rely on group-level data from cross-sectional studies, applying these findings to individuals. However, these approaches are fraught with challenges; people with the same disorders can exhibit vastly different symptoms and responses.[5,6] Consequently, there is considerable variability in how individuals within the same diagnostic category present symptoms, with each person potentially exhibiting a unique set of symptoms. Moreover, even among individuals with similar clinical presentations, the underlying network structures of these symptoms can differ significantly.[7,8] This highlights the complexity and individuality of symptom manifestation in psychiatric diagnoses.

If research does not account for individual trajectories and characteristic differences, these unique aspects may be obscured in group-level analyses. This issue arises particularly when studies focus predominantly on mean values, such as in randomized control trials, leading to the oversight of variability between participants. This variability is often mistakenly treated as mere statistical noise, causing the loss of valuable insights into individual behavioral patterns. For instance, while a higher level of avoidance might decrease negative affect in some individuals, it could conversely increase it in others.[9] Therefore, it is crucial to consider individual data to fully understand the diverse trajectories and identify specific differences that hold clinical significance.[10] This individual-focused approach is key to uncovering nuanced understandings of psychological phenomena.

Moreover, the application of collective findings to individual trajectories is contingent upon highly restrictive and often unrealistic assumptions. These include the notion that the process being studied is stationary, meaning that its mean value and variance remain constant over time, and homogeneous, implying that all individuals conform to the same dynamic model. Such assumptions do not align well with the nature of living systems, which are inherently dynamic and diverse.[11,12] In practice, these assumptions are frequently violated in the realms of psychological testing and treatment research.[13] Despite this, a significant portion of clinical psychology still depends on probabilistic, group-level analyses to investigate mechanisms and understand psychopathology, often at the expense of capturing the complex, individualized nature of these phenomena.

Therefore, given the significant heterogeneity both between and within individuals, and the challenges in applying group-level findings to individual cases, there is a pressing need for dynamic, individual-level analyses that embrace this variability.[14,15] Such analyses involve closely examining the symptoms of each individual at multiple time points, followed by tailored, person-specific evaluations. This approach to studying psychopathology acknowledges and dissects the unique mechanisms driving and sustaining each individual's symptomatology. By conducting analyses at this granular level, we can then extrapolate broader, nomothetic generalizations that are more representative and insightful for the collective. This method is crucial for a comprehensive and nuanced understanding of the mechanisms underlying change in mental health.

A NEW APPROACH TO STUDYING CHANGE

The emergence of the so-called "third wave" approaches of cognitive behavioral therapy (CBT) in the 2000s aimed to explore the underlying processes of change in CBT. This sparked debates within the field and expanded the range of intervention strategies. There has been a renewed focus on understanding the central processes of change and studying mediators and moderators, leading to a refocusing of CBT toward processes of changes and away from syndromal disorders. This includes recognizing the importance of philosophic assumptions in intervention methods (eg, relational frame theory in acceptance and commitment therapy and logical positivism in CBT) and emphasizing the need for training in the philosophy of science.

As an answer to these challenges, process-based therapy (PBT) has emerged as a new direction in CBT.[16] It shifts the focus from syndromes to evidence-based processes linked with procedures, encompassing core competencies shared across various CBT approaches. PBT integrates a broader spectrum of concepts and methods, paving the way for a more inclusive, evidence-based approach to behavior change. As attention pivots toward change processes, mental health care transcends disorder-focused models, embracing a holistic approach to psychological well-being. Personalized and precision medicine principles are increasingly applied, paving the way for a future where evidence-based therapy is synonymous with PBT. This marks a significant transformation in the field, promising a more tailored, effective, and person-centered approach to intervention science.

The field has matured sufficiently to revisit Gordon Paul's vision.[17] The authors propose that the time is ripe for modern psychotherapy and intervention science to concentrate on a new fundamental query: "What core biopsychosocial processes should be addressed in this context, with this client, for this goal, and how can they be most efficiently and effectively altered?" This forms the essence of PBT—a context-specific use of evidence-based processes tied to evidence-based procedures, tailored to individuals for problem-solving and well-being enhancement. Unlike treatments centered on syndromes, PBT hones in on theoretically driven, empirically supported processes underpinning positive change, signifying a pivotal shift for the future of evidence-based care.

It is crucial to distinguish between therapeutic processes (fundamental change mechanisms leading to desired treatment outcomes) and therapeutic procedures (methods applied by therapists to achieve agreed-upon goals). Therapy often targets multiple goals, ranked by priority, immediacy, or complexity. At the psychological level, we can understand processes as sequences of biopsychosocial events in domains such as affect, cognition, attention, self, motivation, overt behavior, biophysiology, or sociocultural characteristics that lead to desired changes.[16] Therapeutic processes need to be theory-grounded, dynamic, progressive, and multilevel changes occurring in predictable, empirically established sequences, oriented toward desired outcomes. They are theory-based with falsifiable predictions, dynamic due to potential feedback loops, progressive for long-term success, and multilevel as some processes take precedence over others. Importantly, they address both immediate and long-term objectives. While a therapeutic process is sometimes used broadly to denote the patient-therapist relationship, the authors employ it in a more specific sense, requiring a clearly defined, testable theory meeting empirical standards.

A Complex Network Approach to Psychopathology

The complex network approach to conceptualizing psychopathology is an alternative to the traditional ways of understanding mental disorders.[18] Instead of viewing symptoms as manifestations of an underlying disease, this approach sees symptoms as constitutive of the disorder itself. In other words, psychopathology is not caused by symptoms that reflect a latent disorder, but rather it is the interaction and self-reinforcing system of problems that constitute the psychopathology.[18–20] According to this perspective, a stressful event, for example, does not activate a latent condition like depression, which then leads to the emergence of symptoms. Instead, the event triggers certain problems, which in turn activate other problems. When a sufficient number of problems occur and are connected in a way that maintains the psychopathology, a diagnosable episode of the disorder may be identified. To avoid implying that symptoms indicate the presence of an underlying disease, the authors prefer the term "problem" instead of "symptom." Psychopathology is seen as functionally interconnected problems that form a complex network.

Network theory is a subset of graph theory, which is a branch of mathematics that deals with visually representing a group of objects and the connections between them. Networks consist of nodes (ie, problems, aspects of suffering), and edges, which are the lines connecting 2 nodes and represent the type of association between them. In an unweighted network, the presence or absence of a line between 2 nodes indicates whether they are connected. On the other hand, a weighted network not only shows the connection but also represents the strength of association, such as using a Pearson r correlation coefficient to indicate the magnitude of association between insomnia and fatigue calculated across multiple individuals. The network structure provides information about what a problem consists of and what sustains it. Network dynamics also provide information on how processes develop and can be changed over time.

Centrality metrics in network theory allow us to determine the relative importance of a node within a network.[21] A highly central node is one that, when activated, has the potential to spread activation throughout the network via its connections to other nodes. For instance, a node with high-degree centrality is one that is connected to many other nodes, similar to a highly popular person in a social network. On the other hand, a node with high-strength centrality in a weighted network is characterized by having connections with large magnitudes of associations, such as edges with a high Pearson's r value. Lastly, a node with high-betweenness centrality often lies on the shortest path between 2 other nodes, acting as a mediator or connector within the network.

Complex networks are characterized by nodes that are interconnected in a nonrandom and nonuniform manner.[22] This means that some nodes form clusters or subgroups, while others have fewer or weaker connections. Such complex networks are commonly observed in fields like sociology, neuroscience, and psychopathology. By repeatedly assessing the nodes and connections in a network, we can observe how the network evolves over time, which is often referred to as network dynamics. This can be seen in the trajectory, or recovery, from psychopathology.

The diagnostic implications of the network perspective are focused on understanding psychopathology in a new way rather than providing a new method of diagnosis. Instead of replacing the DSM or the International Statistical Classification of Diseases and Related Health Problems systemICD, the network perspective offers a fresh perspective on the ontology of psychopathology. It shifts the focus toward identifying the defining features of the pathology (nodes) and their functional connections (edges), rather than searching for a common underlying cause expressed as a sum score of severity. In this approach, the emphasis is on investigating the mechanisms or biomarkers that cause specific elements of the disorder, such as anhedonia, rather than diagnosing the overall disorder itself, such as major depression.

The network perspective on diagnoses recognizes that there are different patterns of symptoms within a diagnostic category, which is different from how the DSM has traditionally viewed heterogeneity. Instead of considering heterogeneity as separate underlying factors within a diagnosis, each with its own cause, the network perspective sees heterogeneity as common patterns that indicate causal connections between different features of a disorder. For example, the network perspective may consider the relationship between the diurnal variation of mood and early morning awakening in the context of the melancholic network.

The network perspective provides a unique approach to differential diagnosis. Instead of simply determining whether a fear of driving is caused by specific phobia or posttraumatic stress disorder, the focus should be on understanding the active symptoms/problems and how they relate to each other. This approach is similar to the functional analysis used by behavior therapists, which examines the links between environmental stimuli and symptoms. However, the network perspective considers the functional relations between a large number of different nodes, not just between 2 variables. The complex network approach also offers the possibility of integrating the multidimensional facets of psychopathology,[18,19] which should prove advantageous given the biopsychosocial nature of psychopathology.[23,24] For example, psychopathologic, psychological, and biological processes that influence psychopathology and their interrelationships can be conceptualized together.

It should be noted that a network approach resolves the comorbidity problem in psychiatry. Traditional diagnostic efforts have focused on eliminating nonspecific symptoms that are present in multiple disorders, in order to distinguish between comorbid disorders. The network analytical framework recognizes the importance of these nonspecific elements and views them as crucial connections. When activated, these connections transmit activation to features of several related disorders.[25]

Critical Role of Causality

Dynamic networks offer a promising approach for studying such treatment processes, as they can provide insight into the causal relationships between variables.[26] Prevention and therapy can only be implemented efficiently if it is clear which variables are causally linked to each other. The inference of causal relationships can be understood as the ability to modify the probability distribution of 1 problem caused by the presence or alteration, whether experimental or natural, of another problem.[19] However, in order to understand causalities in psychological phenomena, it is not only relevant to describe **whether** 1 variable influences another, but also to explain **how** this change comes about,[27] which ultimately leads to the study of mechanisms. The investigation of mechanisms requires more than the mere description of cause-and-effect relationships. The context—other involving variables and the environment—plays a crucial role. For example, a variable such as a spark may be causal for an effect such as an explosion in a silo, but only under specific conditions, such as in the presence of dust and oxygen. In the psychological domain, mechanisms are also links between problems, but they depend on other problems involved and the context, as these factors are also largely responsible for changes.

To identify causal mechanisms of change, temporal knowledge regarding the relationship between problems is essential. There is much debate about whether causal inference is also possible using cross-sectional data.[28,29] However, structural modeling strategies applied to cross-sectional data usually still require temporal knowledge regarding temporal precedence and causal ordering, which by nature can only arise from temporal data. Temporal precedence is a necessary condition for causal inference, making dynamic analyses essential at any point in the inference process, as only these can estimate the directionality of edges.[30,31] Inferences based on cross-sectional data are not the same as those based on longitudinal data and do not reveal how problems influence each other over time.[32] Furthermore, psychopathology is not stable over time,[33,34] which makes multiple measurements over time necessary to reflect this discontinuity.

By determining the direction of the relationships through multiple measurements over time, it is possible to identify and distinguish between primary causal symptoms and epiphenomena. Epiphenomena are secondary phenomena that are not causally related to the primary causal symptom, but may appear to be correlated. It can therefore be an effect of the primary symptom or other underlying factors, but not itself have an effect on the primary symptom or others. The detection of epiphenomena is relevant in that they may represent a distinct condition, but do not themselves play a role in maintaining mechanisms. For example, loss of interest, as 1 of several problems of a patient, may be comparatively relevant and stressful for the patient. By examining the temporal dependencies among all problems, it may become evident that this problem is reinforced by 1 or more other problems (eg, listlessness, reduced mood).

However, in this case, it may not exert influence on other problems, thereby playing a comparatively minor role in maintaining the overall problem—it is not causally responsible for other problem areas, which makes it an epiphenomenon. While loss of interest may initially seem relevant, it might be advisable in this case to prioritize addressing other influential problems. Understanding temporal dependencies therefore allows for the differentiation between variables that have a causal effect in a complex of problems and those that are coincidental or influenced by other factors.

Studying Processes of Change

The ability to identify signals that predict transitions from nonpathologic states to pathologic states and vice versa is particularly valuable to clinical scientists. For this, experience sampling methods,[35] also known as ecological momentary assessment (EMA),[36] will be critically important. The use of EMA in studying psychopathology represents a significant shift toward understanding mental disorders in real-time and real-world contexts.[37] Just as people's well-being fluctuates in response to their environment and daily experiences, so too does their psychological state in the context of psychopathology.[38] These moment-to-moment experiences are crucial in understanding the dynamic nature of psychopathology. Traditional methods, which often rely on retrospective or global assessments, can miss the nuanced changes and patterns that occur in the daily lives of individuals with psychopathology.[39] EMA allows researchers to move beyond these limitations, adopting a dynamic modeling approach to capture how symptoms and their interactions change across different contexts and over time.

The proliferation of mobile health (mHealth) tools has significantly impacted the study of psychopathology, particularly in the collection of EMA data. The use of mHealth tools in EMA data collection is pivotal in enhancing the design and implementation of psychopathology interventions[38] making these programs more accessible and sustainable for a wider range of individuals. Furthermore, mHealth tools facilitate the gathering of intensive longitudinal data, involving numerous measurements over time from a significant number of individuals. This approach allows for the observation of time-structured patterns in symptomatology, providing a deeper understanding of how these momentary changes contribute to the overall trajectory of a mental disorder. Studies in this area, such as those by Kuppens and colleagues[40] have identified 3 specific components of dynamical change that are sufficient for describing individual differences in time-varying patterns: (1) changes in baseline, reflecting long-term shifts in a person's average psychological experience and indicating whether these changes are trending positively, negatively, or remaining stable; (2) intraindividual variability (IIV), which captures the extent and nature of fluctuation in a person's psychological experiences on a momentary level; and (3) regulation, focusing on the rate at which individuals return to their baseline levels of experience, thereby measuring the speed and efficiency of psychological regulation following deviations. Together, these components provide a comprehensive understanding of how momentary changes contribute to the overall trajectory of a mental disorder, offering valuable insights into individual differences in time-varying patterns of psychopathology.[40]

These dynamic characteristics of psychological patterns can be effectively mapped onto various statistical process model parameters. This includes time series and differential equation model parameters, as explored in the work of Hamaker and colleagues.[33] By applying these models, researchers can quantitatively analyze and interpret the complex dynamics of psychological experiences over time. This approach allows for a more nuanced analysis of psychopathology, moving beyond static assessments to capture the fluid and evolving nature of psychological experiences. Moreover, this methodology can aid in the development of personalized treatment strategies. By identifying specific patterns of emotional change and regulation in individuals, clinicians can tailor interventions to address the unique dynamics of each person's psychopathology. This personalized approach is crucial for effective treatment, as it considers the individual variability and complexity inherent in mental health disorders.

NOVEL METHODOLOGY AND STATISTICAL ANALYSIS
Dynamic Network Analysis

Dynamic network analysis is a methodological approach that delves into the intricacies of complex systems. Importantly, this framework provides a systematic and mathematical principled way to model how change in 1 variable (ie, node) affects other variables in the network, and further, how change in the whole or part of the network is related to the strength of the connections and the overall geometry of the network.

The true power of dynamic network analysis lies in its ability to reveal how changes in 1 part of the network (a single node or a group of nodes) can influence the entire network. For instance, an increase in a specific symptom might lead to changes in other symptoms, reflecting the interconnected nature of psychological states. The analysis also considers the overall structure and geometry of the network, which can provide insights into how robust or vulnerable the network is to changes in specific nodes. For example, a network with many strong interconnections might be more resilient to change in any single node, compared to a network with fewer or weaker connections.

Furthermore, dynamic network analysis can identify central nodes that have a significant impact on the network. These central nodes might be key symptoms or factors that, when addressed in treatment, could lead to broader improvements across the network. By understanding these dynamics, clinicians and researchers can develop more targeted and effective interventions for psychopathology, tailored to the specific network dynamics of an individual or a group. This approach marks a significant shift from traditional methods, offering a more nuanced and comprehensive understanding of the complex interplay of factors in mental health and illness.

Networks are used in the study of clinical disorders and comorbidity,[18,20,41] cognition and intelligence,[42] personality,[43] and many others.[44] Within the framework of psychological well-being for instance, network modeling has been used to examine elements of psychological well-being as an interconnected network in early adulthood[45] and further to examine distinctions among measures of well-being.[46]

Control Theory

Importantly, from a mathematical standpoint, dynamic network models are closely related to network control theory,[47] the engineering study of network systems under intervention. Control theory models the dynamics of complex systems and analyzes functional relationships, resilience, and control of the system.[47–49] It enables the quantitative assessment and prediction about the reaction of the entire network and its nodes to both endogenous and exogenous input signals and dynamics over time, and identifies nodes that control the organization of the system.[50,51] The controllability of a network refers to the ability to manipulate network components in order to control the system along a desired trajectory, that is, to bring it to a desired target state. Therefore, it allows for the investigation and evaluation of the effects of psychological interventions on the overall condition of an individual.[51] The ability of a network node to control the rest of the system can be described by the metrics average controllability,[52] modal controllability,[53] and boundary controllability.[50]

Control theory combined with longitudinal data not only provides a comprehensive understanding of the changes in networked systems but also identifies the mechanisms of change driving psychological interventions and their relation to system changes.[54,55] Hypotheses about mechanisms of change can be tested experimentally using network control theory. As an example, this methodology has been used to study the effect of an attitude modification intervention through a dynamic network and control approach.[51] Using dynamic network modeling, the relationship between topological network features and alterations in the network were examined over time. This study demonstrated that intervention effects can be tested using dynamic network models with unparalleled accuracy.[51]

Group Iterative Multiple Model Estimation

The analysis of mechanisms at the individual level is essential, as the mechanisms responsible for changes differ from 1 individual to another. However, for a comprehensive scientific understanding, it's equally important to derive general principles that acknowledge these individual differences. Such generalizations are key in identifying broader patterns and connections that transcend individual cases. This approach lays the groundwork for creating more inclusive models and intervention strategies, ensuring they are both broadly applicable and sensitive to individual variations.

A statistical method to gain a deeper understanding of mechanisms is the group iterative multiple model estimation (GIMME).[56] GIMME uses unified structural equation modeling[57] to initially identify unique associations between symptoms for each individual. Assuming that individuals have similar representations of causal structures, it then iteratively integrates pathways that are applicable at the group levels if they improve individual fit.[58] This approach diverges from traditional methods that view individual variability as an error in estimating group-level central tendencies. Instead, GIMME estimates individual models based on IIV, subsequently generalizing these findings nomothetically. By integrating causal structures from both individual and group levels, GIMME facilitates more effective and precise generalizations about common mechanisms within the target population.[59]

GIMME considers temporal dependencies between variables and thus provides insights into the temporal precedence and directionality of the associations between variables at individual, subgroup, and group levels.[60] The temporal dimension improves the understanding of how symptoms unfold and potentially have a causal effect on the overall disorder (eg, captured by network analyses). This contributes to a deeper understanding of complex systems and their underlying mechanisms.

SUMMARY

The latent disease model of psychiatry, while foundational, has shown limitations in addressing the complex, interconnected nature of psychopathology. The examination of therapeutic change has evolved, moving beyond linear models to embrace more nuanced methods that provide idiographic considerations as well as the dynamic interplay of symptoms over time. The role of the individual in understanding and treating psychopathology has become a focus of research, underscoring the need for personalized approaches that account for the unique symptom networks of each person.

Subsequently, the emergence of PBT marks a significant shift in CBT, focusing on processes rather than syndromal disorders. PBT is built upon the complex network approach to psychopathology which provides a fresh perspective on mental disorders, viewing them as systems of interconnected problems rather than manifestations of an underlying disease. Therapy as a dynamic system highlights the importance of understanding the resilience and control of psychological networks as well as the causal pathways present. This perspective, in turn, can be crucial for developing interventions that effectively target pathways through which networks can be shifted toward healthier states. While researchers have begun examining the therapeutic programs through a dynamic systems approach, further empirical work is needed to provide evidence for this approach. This article underscores the importance of moving beyond traditional models and embracing more dynamic, individual-focused approaches to better understand and treat psychopathology and promote mental health.

CLINICS CARE POINTS

- A network approach allows for a more comprehensive view of the client's problems.
- Process-based therapy provides tailored an person-oriented care.
- One of the challenges of PBT is the standardization of the approach for therapists from different theoretical orientations.

DISCLOSURE

The authors of this article have no conflict of interest to disclose. Dr S.G. Hofmann receives financial support from the Alexander von Humboldt Foundation (as part of the Alexander von Humboldt Professur) and the Hessische Ministerium für Wissenschaft und Kunst (as part of the LOEWE Spitzenprofessur). He also receives compensation for his work as an editor from Springer Nature and royalties and payments for his work from various publishers. Funding received from he Hessian Ministry of Education and Art.

REFERENCES

1. American Psychiatric Association. Diagnostic and statistical manual of mental disorders fifth edition DSM-5. Washington, DC: APA Press; 2013.
2. Baron RM, Kenny DA. The moderator–mediator variable distinction in social psychological research: Conceptual, strategic, and statistical considerations. J Pers Soc Psychol 1986;51:1173–82.
3. Van Noorden R, Maher B, Nuzzo R. The top 100 papers. Nature 2014;514(7524): 550–3.
4. Hofmann SG, Curtiss JE, Hayes SC. Beyond linear mediation: Toward a dynamic network approach to study treatment processes. Clin Psychol Rev 2020;76: 101824.
5. Contractor AA, Roley-Roberts ME, Lagdon S, et al. Heterogeneity in patterns of DSM-5 posttraumatic stress disorder and depression symptoms: Latent profile analyses. J Affect Disord 2017;212:17–24.
6. Fried EI, Nesse RM. Depression is not a consistent syndrome: An investigation of unique symptom patterns in the STAR*D study. J Affect Disord 2015;172:96–102.
7. Galatzer-Levy IR, Bryant RA. 636,120 Ways to Have Posttraumatic Stress Disorder. Perspect Psychol Sci 2013;8(6):651–62.
8. Woods WC, Arizmendi C, Gates KM, et al. Personalized Models of Psychopathology as Contextualized Dynamic Processes: An Example from Individuals with Borderline Personality Disorder. J Consult Clin Psychol 2020;88(3):240–54.

9. Brockman R, Ciarrochi J, Parker P, et al. Emotion regulation strategies in daily life: mindfulness, cognitive reappraisal and emotion suppression. Cogn Behav Ther 2017;46(2):91–113.

10. Barlow DH, Nock MK, Hersen M. Single case experimental designs: strategies for studying behavior for change. 3rd edition. Boston, MA: Pearson/Allyn and Bacon; 2009.

11. Molenaar PCM. On the implications of the classical ergodic theorems: Analysis of developmental processes has to focus on intra-individual variation. Dev Psychobiol 2008;50:60–9.

12. Peters O. The ergodicity problem in economics. Nat Phys 2019;15(12):1216–21.

13. Gomes CMA, de Araujo J, do Nascimento E, et al. Routine Psychological Testing of the Individual Is Not Valid. Psychol Rep 2019;122(4):1576–93.

14. Fisher AJ, Medaglia JD, Jeronimus BF. Lack of group-to-individual generalizability is a threat to human subjects research. Proc Natl Acad Sci USA 2018; 115(27):E6106–15.

15. Wright AGC, Woods WC. Personalized models of psychopathology. Annu Rev Clin Psychol 2020;16:49–74.

16. Hofmann SG, Hayes SC. The future of intervention science: process-based therapy. Clin Psychol Sci 2019;7(1):37–50.

17. Paul GL. Behavior modification research: design and tactics. In: Franks CM, editor. Behavior therapy: appraisal and status. New York City, NY: McGraw-Hill; 1969. p. 29–62.

18. Hofmann SG, Curtiss J, McNally RJ. A complex network perspective on clinical science. Perspect Psychol Sci 2016;11(5):597–605.

19. Borsboom D. A network theory of mental disorders. World Psychiatr 2017; 16(1):5–13.

20. Borsboom D, Cramer AOJ. Network analysis: an integrative approach to the structure of psychopathology. Annu Rev Clin Psychol 2013;9:91–121.

21. Bringmann LF, Elmer T, Epskamp S, et al. What do centrality measures measure in psychological networks? J Abnorm Psychol 2019;128(8):892–903.

22. Barabasi AL, Albert R. Emergence of scaling in random networks. Science 1999; 286(5439):509–12.

23. Astill Wright L, Roberts NP, Barawi K, et al. Disturbed Sleep Connects Symptoms of Posttraumatic Stress Disorder and Somatization: A Network Analysis Approach. J Trauma Stress 2021;34(2):375–83.

24. Tao Y, Hou W, Niu H, et al. Centrality and bridge symptoms of anxiety, depression, and sleep disturbance among college students during the COVID-19 pandemic—a network analysis. Curr Psychol 2022. https://doi.org/10.1007/s12144-022-03443-x.

25. Jones PJ, Ma R, McNally RJ. Bridge Centrality: A Network Approach to Understanding Comorbidity. Multivariate Behav Res 2021;56(2):353–67.

26. Schmittmann VD, Cramer AOj, Waldorp LJ, et al. Deconstructing the construct: A network perspective on psychological phenomena. New Ideas Psychol 2013; 31(1):43–53.

27. Kazdin AE. Mediators and mechanisms of change in psychotherapy research. Annu Rev Clin Psychol 2007;3:1–27.

28. Wunsch G, Russo F, Mouchart M. Do We Necessarily Need Longitudinal Data to Infer Causal Relations? BMS: Bulletin of Sociological Methodology / Bulletin de Méthodologie Sociologique. 2010;106:5–18.

29. Savitz DA, Wellenius GA. Can Cross-Sectional Studies Contribute to Causal Inference? It Depends. Am J Epidemiol 2023;192(4):514–6.

30. Thoemmes F. Reversing Arrows in Mediation Models Does Not Distinguish Plausible Models. Basic Appl Soc Psychol 2015;37(4):226–34.
31. Bringmann LF, Vissers N, Wichers M, et al. A network approach to psychopathology: new insights into clinical longitudinal data. PLoS One 2013;8(4):e60188.
32. Bos FM, Snippe E, Vos S de, et al. Can We Jump from Cross-Sectional to Dynamic Interpretations of Networks Implications for the Network Perspective in Psychiatry. PPS 2017;86(3):175–7.
33. Hamaker EL, Ceulemans E, Grasman RPPP, et al. Modeling affect dynamics: State of the art and future challenges. Emotion Review 2015;7:316–22.
34. Heshmati S, DavyRomano E, Chow C, et al. Negative emodiversity is associated with emotional eating in adolescents: An examination of emotion dynamics in daily life. J Adolesc 2023;95(1):115–30.
35. Csikszentmihalyi M, Larson R. Validity and reliability of the experience-sampling method. J Nerv Ment Dis 1987;175(9):526–36.
36. Shiffman S, Stone AA, Hufford MR. Ecological momentary assessment. Annu Rev Clin Psychol 2008;4:1–32.
37. Heshmati S, Kibrislioglu Uysal N, Kim SH, et al. Momentary PERMA: An Adapted Measurement Tool for Studying Well-Being in Daily Life. J Happiness Stud 2023. https://doi.org/10.1007/s10902-023-00684-w.
38. Heshmati S, Muth C, Li Y, et al. Capturing the Heterogenous Effects of a Mobile-Health Psychological Well-Being Intervention for Early Adults: Results from a Process-Oriented Approach, 2023. https://doi.org/10.31234/osf.io/mb79u.
39. Gorin AA, Stone AA. Recall biases and cognitive errors in retrospective self-reports: a call for momentary assessments. In: Baum A, Revenson T, Singer J, editors. Handbook of Health Psychology. Mahwah, NJ: Erlbaum; 2001. p. 405–14.
40. Kuppens P, Oravecz Z, Tuerlinckx F. Feelings change: accounting for individual differences in the temporal dynamics of affect. J Pers Soc Psychol 2010;99(6): 1042–60.
41. McNally RJ, Mair P, Mugno BL, et al. Co-morbid obsessive-compulsive disorder and depression: a Bayesian network approach. Psychol Med 2017;47(7): 1204–14.
42. Schmank CJ, Goring SA, Kovacs K, et al. Psychometric Network Analysis of the Hungarian WAIS. J Intell 2019;7(3):21.
43. Christensen AP, Golino H, Silvia PJ. A Psychometric Network Perspective on the Validity and Validation of Personality Trait Questionnaires. Eur J Pers 2020;34(6): 1095–108.
44. Westaby JD, Pfaff DL, Redding N. Psychology and social networks: A dynamic network theory perspective. Am Psychol 2014;69(3):269–84.
45. Heshmati S, Oravecz Z, Brick TR, et al. Assessing psychological well-being in early adulthood: Empirical evidence for the structure of daily well-being via network analysis. Appl Dev Sci 2022;26(2):207–25.
46. Merritt SH, Heshmati S, Oravecz Z, Donaldson SI. Web of well-being: Re-examining PERMA and subjective well-being through networks. J Posit Psychol 2023;1–11.
47. Liu YY, Slotine JJ, Barabási AL. Controllability of complex networks. Nature 2011; 473(7346):167–73.
48. Hyland ME. Control theory interpretation of psychological mechanisms of depression: Comparison and integration of several theories. Psychol Bull 1987;102: 109–21.
49. Liu YY, Barabási AL. Control principles of complex systems. Rev Mod Phys 2016; 88(3):035006.

50. Hahn T, Jamalabadi H, Emden D, et al. A Network Control Theory Approach to Longitudinal Symptom Dynamics in Major Depressive Disorder. Published online July 21, 2021. doi:10.48550/arXiv.2107.10178.
51. Stocker JE, Koppe G, Reich H, et al. Formalizing psychological interventions through network control theory. Sci Rep 2023;13(1):13830.
52. Gu S, Pasqualetti F, Cieslak M, et al. Controllability of structural brain networks. Nat Commun 2015;6(1):8414.
53. Scheffer M. Foreseeing tipping points. Nature 2010;467(7314):411–2.
54. Jamalabadi H, Hofmann SG, Teutenberg L, et al. A complex systems model of temporal fluctuations in depressive symptomatology. Published online December 13, 2023. doi:10.31234/osf.io/fm76b.
55. Wu Y, Mo J, Sui L, et al. Deep Brain Stimulation in Treatment-Resistant Depression: A Systematic Review and Meta-Analysis on Efficacy and Safety. Front Neurosci 2021;15:655412.
56. Gates KM, Molenaar PCM. Group search algorithm recovers effective connectivity maps for individuals in homogeneous and heterogeneous samples. Neuroimage 2012;63(1):310–9.
57. Kim J, Zhu W, Chang L, et al. Unified structural equation modeling approach for the analysis of multisubject, multivariate functional MRI data. Hum Brain Mapp 2007;28:85–93.
58. Lane ST, Gates KM, Pike HK, et al. Uncovering general, shared, and unique temporal patterns in ambulatory assessment data. Psychol Methods 2019;24(1):54–69.
59. Lane ST, Gates KM. Automated Selection of Robust Individual-Level Structural Equation Models for Time Series Data. Struct Equ Model: A Multidiscip J 2017;24(5):768–82.
60. Gates KM, Lane ST, Varangis E, et al. Unsupervised Classification During Time-Series Model Building. Multivariate Behav Res 2017;52(2):129–48.

Cognitive Behavioral Therapy
Strategies for Enhancing Treatment Engagement

Nikolaos Kazantzis, PhD, FAPS, BICBT-CC[a,b,*]

KEYWORDS

- Cognitive behavioral therapy • Treatment engagement • Clinician skill

KEY POINTS

- Patient engagement with homework is pivotal, given the short-term nature of cognitive behavioral therapy (CBT) and its emphasis on cognitive, emotional, behavioral, and interpersonal changes.
- Challenges in patient engagement range from managing competing demands to unexpected clinical matters and activation of negative core beliefs.
- Meta-analytic reviews suggest that homework significantly enhances CBT effectiveness for depression and anxiety disorders.
- Treatment engagement involves both behavioral principles of learning and cognitive determinants, extending beyond traditional behavioral theories.
- The clinician's role is pivotal in fostering engagement, and recent research emphasizes therapist behavior as a significant factor.

INTRODUCTION

Treatment engagement, defined as the consistent implementation of negotiated between-session therapy tasks (homework), stands as one of the most influential factors shaping outcomes in cognitive behavioral therapy (CBT).[1,2] This assertion is substantiated by two lines of reasoning. Firstly, given its nature as a short-term psychological therapy model emphasizing cognitive, emotional, behavioral, and interpersonal changes, the patient's active involvement with homework emerges as a pivotal aspect of the therapeutic process. Secondly, a convergence of evidence from experimental research, which compares therapy with and without homework, correlational studies investigating the relationship between homework adherence/

[a] Cognitive Behavior Therapy Research Unit, PO Box 515, Collins Street, Melbourne, Victoria 8007 Australia; [b] Beck Institute for Cognitive Behavior Therapy, Philadelphia, PA, USA
* Cognitive Behavior Therapy Research Unit, PO Box 515, Collins Street, Melbourne, Victoria 8007 Australia.
E-mail address: admin@cbtru.com

Psychiatr Clin N Am 47 (2024) 301–310
https://doi.org/10.1016/j.psc.2024.03.002
0193-953X/24/© 2024 Elsevier Inc. All rights reserved.

compliance and outcomes, and field surveys involving clinicians in diverse practice settings uniformly underscores the significance of patient engagement in CBT.[3–6]

This article begins with an overview of the clinical features associated with departures from consistent engagement during therapy sessions, followed by a review of empirical evidence supporting the crucial role of homework adherence/compliance in CBT. Acknowledging the variability in patient engagement with clinician-negotiated recommendations for between-session work, this article provides an overview of the CBT model of treatment engagement. Lastly, practical clinical insights are presented to guide clinicians through frequently encountered scenarios in their practice.

DISCUSSION
Clinical Features

Challenges in patient engagement with therapeutic tasks exist along a continuum, ranging from occasional difficulties managing competing demands to unanticipated practical obstacles in task implementation, unexpected clinical matters arising during task engagement, including the activation of higher-than-anticipated or different types of psychological distress, and salient beliefs about the self, clinician, or the therapy process.[7,8] Adverse effects for the patient are a tangible possibility, particularly given that homework requires the individual to engage in therapeutic strategies without supervision, often involving tasks that contradict existing coping strategies. Two broad categories can be delineated for the lack of or partial completion of therapeutic homework.

Competing demands

This encompasses challenges related to managing psychosocial stressors, especially those involving time demands, organization, or multiple relationships that intensify psychological distress, subsequently exacerbating the presenting disorder. For instance, a patient with depressed mood with high standards for their work may keenly feel the inability to meet these standards in various life areas, activating a theme of failure, especially if therapy tasks are perceived as excessively burdensome. Alternatively, patients may not fully comprehend tasks introduced during sessions, necessitate more practice to develop the required skills for initial implementation, lack insight into their current level of skill acquisition, or be unwilling to provide accurate feedback on their understanding or belief in the between-session work.

Activation of the patient's belief system

Commonly referred to as the overlay of negative core beliefs, this category involves the patient's attitudes toward the clinician and/or the therapeutic process. For instance, if an anxious patient experiences unexpectedly high levels of task difficulty or heightened emotions during an assigned exposure task, they may feel annoyed, angry, or suspicious of the clinician's motives, drawing from strained relationships and perceived mistreatment by others. Some patients may view therapy as a passive "treatment" process, expecting change to occur solely within the consultation time. This may reflect a different conceptualization of change, one relying on clinician insight, or a preference and expectation that change is the clinician's responsibility.

The Empirical State of Homework in Cognitive Behavior Therapy

Homework is consistently integrated into CBT protocols,[9] and the benefits of formally negotiated between-session activities have been examined through experimental and quasi-experimental research designs.[10–13] The findings from several meta-analytic reviews indicate that homework significantly enhances the effectiveness of CBT for depression and anxiety disorders.[14,15] However, caution is warranted, as evidence supporting causal effects across the spectrum of disorders is lacking, and further research in other clinical disorders is necessary.

Meta-analyses examining adherence/compliance and outcome relationships suggest a strong and positive correlation, with higher levels of engagement correlating with greater pre–post-treatment symptom reduction.[16,17] Nevertheless, systematic reviews of measures used in studies have primarily focused on quantity, often assessed through single-item ratings, sometimes retrospectively.[18,19] Quality of completion and patient appraisals of the task have been infrequently considered, despite the clear relevance of patient cognitions in CBT.[20,21]

The past two decades have seen clinician guides including case studies[22] exploring the role of homework across various psychotherapeutic models, with suggestions that it may be considered a specific, common factor in therapy.[23,24] However, research on homework in therapies beyond CBT remains limited, with a predominant focus on specific modifications of CBT, such as trauma-focused therapies and dialectical behavior therapy.[5]

A growing body of research examines the translation or implementation of homework in psychotherapeutic practice.[25–28] Large surveys indicate that practitioners with a CBT theoretic orientation and those employing other therapies, including short-term dynamic therapy, routinely incorporate homework into their practice.[29] Similarly, those utilizing technology for therapy delivery or augmentation report regular adoption of homework.

Until recently, there was minimal research on the role of patient beliefs about homework or the clinician's skill in facilitating an in-session process to foster positive task appraisals and high engagement.[30–34] Recent studies, however, demonstrate that a more careful collaboration and negotiation in homework design and planning result in more positive task appraisals in both child and adult depression.[35] Moreover, patient beliefs about homework are shown to be linked to levels of engagement in treatment.[36,37]

In summary, treatment engagement in CBT has undergone extensive study, revealing clear evidence for both causal and correlational relationships with treatment outcomes. Practitioners routinely incorporate homework into their clinical work, with recent research emphasizing the importance of considering patient beliefs throughout the homework process.

The Cognitive Behavioral Account of Treatment Engagement

Although the concept of treatment engagement in CBT predominantly centers on patient appraisals, this inherently incorporates behavioral principles of learning, encompassing both classical and operant conditioning.[38,39] Simply put, a patient will persist in a therapeutic task and endeavor to apply it across various life domains if it proves beneficial, holding promise in the specific areas of clinical focus. Conversely, nonengagement or partial engagement may occasionally signify a task mismatched to the patient in terms of content or difficulty.[40,41]

The behavior of the clinician plays a pivotal role in fostering engagement, with recent process research emphasizing therapist behavior as a significant correlate of patient beliefs regarding the assigned tasks. This paradigm shift moves away from labeling patients as "nonadherent" or "noncompliant," emphasizing that in-session processes are crucial for effective between-session engagement.[11,12,36]

The cognitive behavioral model of treatment engagement extends beyond the original behavioral theory recommendations, incorporating clear cues for homework implementation and specificity in location, duration, timing, and frequency, to now include cognitive aspects.[42] According to this comprehensive theory, the same cognitive determinants influencing engagement in medications and other clinician-recommended health-related behaviors are applicable to homework.

Most social cognition theories focus on assessing the benefits and costs of recommended health behaviors to enhance motivation and intention to engage.[22,24,42] Both short-term and long-term benefits toward treatment goals are emphasized. For instance, tasks inducing discomfort, such as increasing activity for patients with depressed mood, need to yield an immediate, albeit minor, mood improvement. Those engaged in reappraising depressogenic or catastrophizing cognition should experience emotional relief through more realistic thinking, fostering the belief that patients can actively contribute to positive changes in their situation and may even develop their own homework based on early success experiences.

The potential range and scope of homework tasks are considerable, each with a distinct focus.[43-45] For example, a thought record can aid patients in identifying relevant thoughts, prioritizing thoughts based on emotions, evaluating thoughts based on evidence, or engaging in cognitive reappraisal. The focus of a thought record may also extend to verbal or visual cognitions, facilitating various treatment processes such as emotion identification and coping, acceptance and distancing, and support for interpersonal skill training.

Fig. 1 illustrates the nested targets and uses for CBT techniques, providing a visual representation of the core considerations in determining the rationale and benefits of a CBT homework task for a patient.

When applied to individual patients, careful consideration of the precise meaning and interpretation of the task becomes necessary, taking into account their idiosyncratic beliefs regarding problems and coping strategies, which may, to some extent, reflect personality traits. For example, a patient struggling with self-discipline might hold a preconceived notion that a task is likely to be unsuccessful, interpreting any

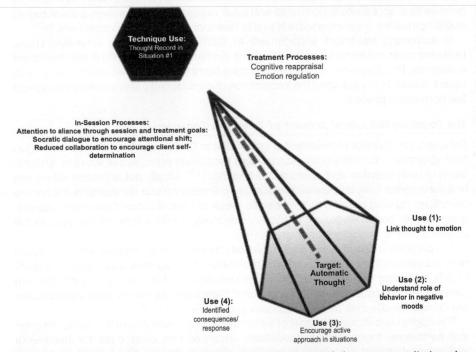

Fig. 1. The process model of techniques in cognitive behavioral therapy as applied to the thought record. (*From* Kazantzis, N. "Introduction to the Special Issue on Processes of Cognitive Behavioral Therapy: Does 'Necessary, But Not Sufficient' Still Capture It?" Cogn Ther Res 42, 115–120 (2018). https://doi.org/10.1007/s10608-018-9891-z); with permission.)

lack of progress as part of a broader pattern in attempts toward self-help or adopting a healthy lifestyle. On the other hand, a patient who tends to avoid expressing emotions may face additional challenges in recognizing the incremental benefits of a given task. Therefore, the process of selecting tasks should ideally be collaborative, with the patient's experience serving as the metric for evaluation. Specific hypotheses are generated, and the identification of beliefs involves a Socratic dialogue with the aim of providing new information and supporting the patient in gaining a fresh understanding of how the prescribed homework task may be beneficial.

Two additional processes are crucial for treatment engagement. Firstly, the collaborative process of developing a specific plan includes determining when, where, how often, and for how long the homework should be undertaken. Following a summary that recaps the rationale and ensures the patient's comprehension of the task, the patient can then assess their readiness, perceived importance, and confidence regarding the task. Ideally, the clinician supports the patient in anticipating and problem-solving practical obstacles throughout this process.

Secondly, the collaborative review of homework involves assessing learning outcomes, with a focus on skill acquisition rather than merely the quantity of completed tasks. This review is ideally sequenced at the outset of the subsequent session, allowing any arising clinical matters to be prioritized on the session's agenda, including time for problem-solving practical obstacles and recalibration if the patient perceives the task as excessively challenging. If the patient modifies or selects a different task relevant to their goals, acknowledging independent thinking is essential, and the extent to which the work aligns with therapy goals and proves adaptive should be determined. Adhering to the principles of reinforcement, shaping, and generalization for the maintenance of therapeutic gains, the clinician identifies the patient's perceived progress, mastery of skills, and any enjoyment or relief of emotional strain.

The cognitive behavioral account of treatment engagement is illustrated in **Fig. 2**, highlighting key clinician considerations in the design, planning, and review of homework tasks.

The subsequent sections of the article delve into strategies for addressing common difficulties in facilitating engagement in CBT.

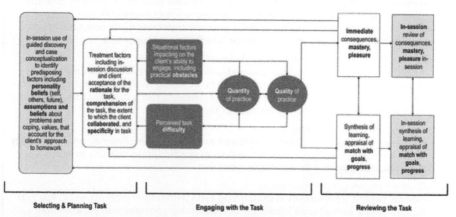

Fig. 2. The comprehensive model of homework in cognitive behavioral therapy. (*From* Kazantzis, N., Miller, A.R. "A Comprehensive Model of Homework in Cognitive Behavior Therapy." Cogn Ther Res 46, 247–257 (2022). https://doi.org/10.1007/s10608-021-10247-z); with permission.)

CLINICS CARE POINTS

- Addressing the perception of "no motivation"
  An indirect yet powerful means of addressing motivation involves defining it as an emotion and placing it on a continuum with patient-defined anchor points, as is customary in CBTs. This allows for the assessment and evaluation of small incremental changes in motivation during sessions, illustrating the pitfalls of binary or "all-or-nothing" thinking about emotions. Informing the patient about the proximity of the memory center and amygdala within the brain, and highlighting the creation of new memories from enjoyable experiences, can result in enhanced motivation. Adjusting expectations for an immediate feeling of motivation to a more realistic anticipation of increased motivation over time, in terms of psychophysiology, is often compelling to patients.[46] Maintaining a motivational interviewing style ensures that patients view tasks as having clear benefits that outweigh the associated time, energy, and sometimes financial implications.

- Addressing "perfectionism"
  Patients identifying as "perfectionists" or holding exceptionally high standards benefit from recognizing their values. Acknowledging the patient's self-concept as someone who achieves or strives for their best effort is crucial. Establishing clear metrics for task assessment, where progress and success can be operationalized, is advantageous. Introducing a "no-lose" task, informative or beneficial regardless of the result, akin to CBT "behavioral experiments," supports the patient in aligning their actions with their value.

- Addressing perceived "low-confidence" to engage
  Patients expressing low confidence often harbor negative core beliefs about themselves, requiring modification early in therapy to facilitate engagement with challenging homework tasks. Recognition of potential negative beliefs stemming from developmental trauma, doubts about self-worth, and anticipation of inconsistent support is crucial. Addressing these beliefs aids in fostering a more constructive therapeutic relationship.

- Addressing perceived judgment from the clinician
  Acknowledging the existence of negative core beliefs and assumptions in patients is essential, especially during highly distressing emotional states or significant psychosocial stressors. Recognizing potential prior experiences of judgment from the health care system or previous clinicians is vital. Providing a supportive, nonjudgmental environment fosters trust and collaboration.

- Addressing "resistance" to change
  Taking an open, collaborative approach that considers the patient's beliefs, values, and preferred working style is an effective stance. Clinicians must be attentive to potential strain in the therapeutic alliance during the integration of homework into therapy.[28] Repairing ruptures in the alliance involves moment-to-moment case conceptualization, considering both the patient's and clinician's beliefs and assumptions.

- Addressing a perception of being "overwhelmed"
  If a patient expresses feeling overwhelmed, adjustments to task demands may be necessary. Collaboration with significant others, including family, and providing periodic feedback during sessions can be beneficial. The clinician's role is to make tasks challenging but not overwhelming, stacking the odds in favor of success.

- Addressing task understanding
  Encourage patients to keep session notes and a summary of task rationale on a technology device to mitigate memory biases.[47,48] In-session practice offers valuable experience, feedback, and guidance for task implementation.

- Addressing challenges in organization
  Patients benefit from support in strategizing tasks within their working week. Practical considerations, such as work conditions or relationship contexts, warrant attention. Providing guidance on task integration and organization is essential for successful implementation.

- Addressing cognitive diversity
  Many of the concepts and tasks in CBT are abstract and may be challenging for patients with cognitive impairment or learning disabilities. Similarly, patients who have high or exceptionally high intelligence may have specific beliefs about their cognition (eg, noting marked variation in memory capacity for areas of less interest leading to an inaccurate negative appraisal). High-intelligence individuals often do not fully understand the diversity of human experiences and may hold the assumption that others are being lazy or disrespectful if they do not have the same problem-solving capacity. In all instances when working with cognitive diversity, the clinician can usually provide psychoeducation, recognize patient strengths, and support the patient in enhancing self-compassion and self-confidence in their abilities.

SUMMARY

Hopefully, it will be clear from this brief clinical review article that the matter of treatment engagement has been subject to considerable theoretic and empirical work in CBT. Perhaps most prominent is the move away from an allocation of responsibility to the patient to the collaborative exchange with the clinician, particularly in the patient's appraisals of the homework that may reflect broader beliefs within the cognitive case conceptualization. As a reflection of this change in emphasis, the research supporting homework has moved to an assessment of patient beliefs about the homework and the therapist's skill in the facilitation of that engagement.

Many challenges are experienced in the process of integrating homework into therapy, especially in the cases of patients with long-standing problems and a long history of highly active negative core beliefs and those with pervasive difficulties in their interpersonal relationships. The nested processes of change add various means of tailoring a specific technique to be assigned as homework, adding further complexity. Many clinicians describe difficulty in effectively implementing this process of therapy, and many patients experience suboptimal therapy. This underscores the importance of specific therapist training and attention to the comprehensive model of homework in CBT.

DISCLOSURE

N. Kazantzis disclosed his royalties from the Guilford Press (Therapeutic Relationship in Cognitive Behavior Therapy; Cognitive and Behavior Theories in Clinical Practice), Routledge (Using Homework Assignments in Cognitive Behavior Therapy); and Springer Nature publishers (CBT: Science into Practice Book Series; Handbook of Homework Assignments in Psychotherapy: Research, Practice, & Prevention). He also disclosed editor stipend from the Association for Behavioral and Cognitive Therapies for his role as the Editor-in-Chief for Cognitive and Behavioral Practice (Elsevier).

REFERENCES

1. Beck AT, Rush J, Shaw B, et al. Cognitive therapy of depression. New York: Guilford Press; 1979.
2. Beck J. Cognitive therapy for challenging problems: what to do when the basics don't work. New York: Guilford; 2011.
3. Dobson KS. A commentary on the science and practice of homework in cognitive-behavioral therapy. Cogn Ther Res 2021;45:303–9.
4. Huibers MJH, Lorenzo-Luaces L, Cuijpers P, et al. On the road to personalized psychotherapy: A research agenda based on cognitive behavior therapy for depression. Front Psychiatry 2021;1:607508.

5. Kazantzis N. Introduction to the special issue on homework in cognitive-behavioral therapy: New clinical psychological science. Cogn Ther Res 2021;45:205–8.

6. Strunk DR. Homework. Cogn Behav Pract 2022;29(3):560–3.

7. Okamoto A, Dattilio FM, Dobson KS, et al. The therapeutic relationship in cognitive–behavioral therapy: Essential features and common challenges. Pract Innovations 2019;2:112–23.

8. Kazantzis N, Arntz AR, Borkovec T, et al. Unresolved issues regarding homework assignments in cognitive and behavioural therapies: an expert panel discussion at AACBT. Behav Change 2010;27(3):119–29.

9. Kazantzis N. Power to detect homework effects in psychotherapy outcome research. J Consult Clin Psychol 2000;68:166–70.

10. Callan JA, Kazantzis N, Park SY, et al. Effects of cognitive behavior therapy homework adherence on outcomes: propensity score analysis. Behav Ther 2019;50(2):285–99.

11. McEvoy PM, Bendlin M, Johnson AR, et al. The relationships among working alliance, group cohesion and homework engagement in group cognitive behaviour therapy for social anxiety disorder. Psychother Res 2024;34(1):54–67.

12. McEvoy PM, Johnson AR, Kazantzis N, et al. Predictors of homework engagement in group CBT for social anxiety: Client beliefs about homework, its consequences, group cohesion, and working alliance. Psychother Res 2023. https://doi.org/10.1080/10503307.2023.2286993.

13. Neimeyer RA, Kazantzis N, Kassler DM, et al. Group cognitive behavior therapy for depression: Outcomes predicted by willingness to engage in homework, compliance with homework, and cognitive restructuring skill acquisition. Cogn Behav Ther 2008;37:199–215.

14. Kazantzis N, Deane FP, Ronan KR. Homework assignments in cognitive and behavioral therapy: A meta-analysis. Clin Psychol Sci Pract 2000;7:189–202.

15. Kazantzis N, Whittington CJ, Dattilio F. Meta-analysis of homework effects in cognitive and behavioral therapy: A replication and extension. Clin Psychol Sci Pract 2010;17(2):144–56.

16. Mausbach BT, Moore R, Roesch S, et al. The relationship between homework compliance and therapy outcomes: an updated meta-analysis. Cogn Ther Res 2010;34(5):429–38.

17. Kazantzis N, Whittington CJ, Zelencich L, et al. Quantity and quality of homework compliance: A meta-analysis of relations with outcome in cognitive behavior therapy. Behav Ther 2016;47:755–72.

18. Kazantzis N, Brownfield NR, Mosely L, et al. Homework in cognitive behavioral therapy: a systematic review of adherence assessment in anxiety and depression (2011-2016). Psychiatr Clin North Am 2017;40(4):625–39.

19. Kazantzis N, Deane F, Ronan KR. Assessing compliance with homework assignments: Review and recommendations for clinical practice. J Clin Psychol 2004;60(6):627–41.

20. Fehm L, Mrose J. Patients' perspective on homework assignments in cognitive-behavioural therapy. Clin Psychol Psychother 2008;15(5):320–8.

21. Kazantzis N, Deane FP, Ronan KR. Homework rating scale – revised (HRS-II). unpublished scale, cognitive behavior therapy research unit, Melbourne, Victoria, Australia. Scale. Available at: www.cbtru.com.

22. Kazantzis N, Deane FP, Ronan KR, et al. Using homework assignments in cognitive behavior therapy. New York: Routledge; 2005.

23. Nelson DL, Castonguay LG, Barwick F. Directions for the integration of homework in practice. In: Kazantzis N, L'Abate L, editors. Handbook of homework

assignments in psychotherapy: research, practice, prevention. New York: Springer Science; 2007. p. 425–44.

24. Ryum T, Bennion M, Kazantzis N. Integrating between-session homework in psychotherapy: A systematic review of immediate in-session and intermediate outcomes. Psychotherapy 2023a;60(3):306–19.

25. Dattilio FM, Kazantzis N, Carr A, et al. Therapists' attitudes towards barriers impeding homework completion in couples and family therapy. J Marital Fam Ther 2011;37(2):121–36.

26. Fehm L, Kazantzis N. Attitudes and use of homework assignments in therapy: a survey of German psychotherapists. Clin Psychol Psychother 2004;11(5):332–43.

27. Kazantzis N, Dattilio FM. Definitions of homework, types of homework, and ratings of the importance of homework among psychologists with cognitive behavior therapy and psychoanalytic theoretical orientations. J Clin Psychol 2010;66(7):1–16.

28. Kazantzis N, Dattilio FM, Shinkfield G, et al. Clinician experiences of homework in couples and family therapy: A survey of perceived impact on the working alliance. Scand J Psychol 2022;64(1):1–9.

29. Kazantzis N, Lampropoulos GL, Deane FP. A national survey of practicing psychologists' use and attitudes towards homework in psychotherapy. J Consult Clin Psychol 2005;73:742–8.

30. Conklin LR, Strunk DR, Cooper AA. Therapist behaviors as predictors of immediate homework engagement in cognitive therapy for depression. Cogn Ther Res 2018;42(1):16–23.

31. Haller E, Watzke B. The role of homework engagement, homework-related therapist behaviors, and their association with depressive symptoms in telephone-based CBT for depression. Cogn Ther Res 2021;45:224–35.

32. Ryum T, Stiles TC, Svartberg M, et al. The effects of therapist competence in assigning homework in cognitive therapy with cluster C personality disorders: Results from a randomized controlled trial. Cogn Behav Pract 2010;17(3):283–9.

33. Ryum T, Svartberg M, Stiles TC. Homework assignments, agenda setting and the therapeutic alliance in cognitive therapy with cluster C personality disorders: Synergetic or antagonistic ingredients? Cogn Ther Res 2022;46(2):448–55.

34. Weck F, Richtberg S, Esch S, et al. The relationship between therapist competence and homework compliance in maintenance cognitive therapy for recurrent depression: Secondary analysis of a randomized controlled trial. Behav Ther 2013;44:162–72.

35. Hildebrand-Burke C, Davey C, Gwini S, et al. Therapist competence, homework engagement, and client characteristics in CBT for youth depression: A study of mediation and moderation in a community-based trial. Psychother Res 2024;34(1):41–53.

36. Yew RY, Dobson KS, Zyphur M, et al. Mediators and moderators of homework-outcome relations in CBT for depression: A study of engagement, therapist skill, and client factors. Cogn Ther Res 2021;45:209–23.

37. Zelencich LM, Kazantzis N, Wong DN, et al. Predictors of homework engagement in CBT adapted for traumatic brain injury: pre/post-injury and therapy process factors. Cogn Ther Res 2020;44(1):40–51.

38. Shelton JL, Ackerman JM. Homework in counseling and psychotherapy; examples of systematic assignments for therapeutic use by mental health professionals. Springfield, IL: Thomas; 1974.

39. Shelton JL, Levy RL. A survey of the reported use of assigned homework activities in contemporary behavior therapy literature. Behav Ther 1981;4:13–4.

40. Willner-Reid J, Whitaker D, Epstein DH, et al. Cognitive-behavioural therapy for heroin and cocaine use: Ecological momentary assessment of homework simplification and compliance. Psychol Psychother 2016;89(3):276–93.

41. Ryum T, Bennion M, Kazantzis N. Homework as a driver of change in psychotherapy. J Clin Psychol 2023. https://doi.org/10.1002/jclp.23627. Advance online publication.
42. Kazantzis N, Miller AR. A comprehensive model of homework in cognitive behavior therapy. Cogn Ther Res 2021. https://doi.org/10.1007/s10608-021-10247-z.
43. Hayes SC, Ciarrochi J, Hofmann SG, et al. Evolving an idionomic approach to processes of change: Towards a unified personalized science of human improvement. Behav Res Ther 2022;156:1–23.
44. Kazantzis N, Hofmann SG. Additional approaches to treatment of depression. JAMA 2019;321(16):1635.
45. Strunk DR, Lorenzo-Luaces L, Huibers MJH, et al. Editorial: contemporary issues in defining the mechanisms of cognitive behavior therapy. Front Psychiatry 2021;12: 1541.
46. Sijercic I, Button ML, Westra HA, et al. The interpersonal context of client motivational language in cognitive-behavioral therapy. Psychotherapy 2016;53(1):13–21.
47. Aizenstros A, Bakker D, Hofmann S, et al. Engagement with smartphone-delivered behavioural activation interventions: a study of the MoodMission smartphone application. Behav Cognit Psychother 2020;1–13. https://doi.org/10.1017/S1352465820000922.
48. Bunnell BE, Nemeth LS, Lenert LA, et al. Barriers associated with the implementation of homework in youth mental health treatment and potential mobile health solutions. Cogn Ther Res 2021;45(2):272–86.

Cognitive Behavioral Therapy for Anxiety and Depression in Children and Adolescents

Orri Smárason, PhD[a],*, Gudmundur Skarphedinsson, PhD[b],
Eric A. Storch, PhD[c]

KEYWORDS

- Anxiety • Depression • Child • Adolescent • CBT • Cognitive therapy
- Behavior therapy

KEY POINTS

- Anxiety disorders are prevalent in children and adolescents.
- Depression is uncommon in younger children but rises sharply in prevalence during adolescence.
- Cognitive behavioral therapy (CBT) for child and adolescent anxiety emphasizes an exposure component and is highly effective.
- CBT for child and adolescent depression emphasizes 3 core strategies: problem-solving, behavioral activation, and cognitive restructuring, and may be most optimal when part of a combined treatment strategy.
- Innovative technology-based approaches may increase personalization and accessibility, improving the effectiveness of child and adolescent CBT.

INTRODUCTION

Anxiety and depression affect as many as one-third of children and adolescents.[1] The prevalence of anxiety disorders in school-aged children has been estimated at 9% to 30%.[1–3] Anxiety disorders are associated with a wide range of impairments and secondary problems, particularly if left untreated,[4,5] including deficits in social, personal, and academic functioning, potentially extending into adolescence and adulthood.[6,7] Further, childhood anxiety disorders increase the risk for depression and substance abuse in later life.[6,8]

---

[a] Department of Child and Adolescent Psychiatry, Landspitali – The National University Hospital of Iceland, Dalbraut 12 105, Reykjavik; [b] Faculty of Psychology, University of Iceland, Sæmundargata 12 102, Reykjavik; [c] Menninger Department of Psychiatry and Behavioral Sciences, Baylor College of Medicine, 1977 Butler Boulevard, Houston, TX 77030, USA
* Corresponding author.
E-mail address: orris@landspitali.is

Psychiatr Clin N Am 47 (2024) 311–323
https://doi.org/10.1016/j.psc.2024.02.002
0193-953X/24/© 2024 Elsevier Inc. All rights reserved.

Depressive disorders are relatively rare in childhood[9] but prevalence rates rise sharply during adolescence and reach levels of up to 20%.[1,10] In childhood, the prevalence rate of depression is about the same for boys and girls. During adolescence, however, girls show about twice the prevalence rate of boys.[11] Not only do more girls have depressive disorders, they are likely to show more symptoms, more severe symptoms, and a greater risk of self-harm and suicidal thoughts.[12] Adolescent depression can persist into adulthood and have significant impairing effects on social, personal, and academic functioning.[13] Depression is associated with an elevated risk of suicidal ideation and attempts.[14] Despite most adolescents recovering from their initial depressive episode, relapse rates are as high as 50% to 70% within 5 years.[15]

From a developmental perspective, early identification and intervention offer the best opportunity to positively impact the trajectory of depressed and anxious children. Evidence-based and developmentally appropriate interventions, such as cognitive behavioral therapy (CBT), are therefore crucial.

ASSESSMENT OF CHILD AND ADOLESCENT ANXIETY AND DEPRESSION

The foundation for successful treatment planning and case conceptualization for child and adolescent anxiety and depression is provided by conducting a thorough and accurate assessment. Clinician-administered instruments, often in the form of semi-structured diagnostic interviews, and parent-report and youth-report questionnaires are employed as a part of comprehensive diagnostic assessment. Ideally, assessments for youth should use multiple methods and multiple informants.[16]

Parent-report and child-report symptom scales provide a continuous measure of severity and often have subscales that align with specific diagnostic categories. They are often short and can be administered repeatedly during treatment to assess progress.[17,18] To determine diagnostic status, however, clinician-administered diagnostic interviews are the most comprehensive, reliable, and valid method.[19,20]

The results of diagnostic assessments and symptom scales should be integrated with developmental history, contextual variables, and key cognitions and behaviors to form a case conceptualization which includes hypotheses about the etiology and maintenance factors relevant to the case, as well as treatment targets.[21] Case conceptualization is regarded as the foundation for the competent practice of CBT.[22]

COGNITIVE BEHAVIORAL THERAPY FOR ANXIETY

CBT for anxiety disorders is based on the merger of 2 theoretic models: behavior therapy, which focuses on direct attempts to reduce anxiety symptoms by altering behavior, and cognitive therapy which emphasizes altering individual appraisals and thinking patterns.[23,24]

Current Evidence

The evidence base for CBT for child and adolescent anxiety disorders is robust.[25,26] Meta-analyses supporting the effectiveness of CBT indicate about a 60% remission rate, surpassing wait-list and attention controls.[25] Programs such as Coping Cat and Cool Kids have gained international recognition and adaptation,[27–29] due to their effectiveness and acceptability. In the Child/Adolescent Anxiety Multimodal Study (CAMS), 60% of participants receiving CBT showed considerable improvement,[30] with most maintaining their treatment gains at the 36-week follow-up.[31] Furthermore, recent meta-analytic findings indicate that CBT alone is not less effective than a selective serotonin reuptake inhibitor (SSRI) or a combination of CBT and SSRI.[32] Emerging research also suggests the applicability of CBT for anxious children as young as

4 years old,[33] with evidence indicating that CBT is superior to other psychosocial treatments for this age group.[34]

Non–disorder-specific CBT, which targets a spectrum of anxiety disorders, may be less effective for social anxiety disorder while its efficacy for other anxiety disorders is well supported in youth.[29,35,36] An analysis of potential predictor and moderator variables within the CAMS revealed that for children diagnosed with primary social anxiety disorder, CBT alone did not significantly outperform pill placebo. Moreover, it was substantially less effective than sertraline alone or in combination with sertraline.[35] Specialized CBT interventions have been developed for children with social anxiety disorders that incorporate social skills training[37] and/or emphasize cognitive and behavioral elements critical in the development and maintenance of social anxiety.[38] These refined treatment approaches have demonstrated CBT effectiveness for this group.[39]

CBT protocols involve parents in treatment to varying degrees. The optimal level of parental involvement in child therapy for anxiety remains an important area for exploration[40] but is likely critical to target mechanisms associated with anxiety maintenance (eg, family accommodation).[41] Parental factors and family environment play an important role in the development, maintenance, and treatment outcomes of childhood anxiety disorders,[42,43] and increased parental involvement has been suggested as an avenue toward increasing treatment effectiveness.[40] A range of family-based CBT approaches, with varying levels of parental involvement, have been developed and assessed.[40] Some such approaches focus exclusively on parents and require no, or very minimal, contact between the child and therapist.[44,45] Evidence suggests that family-based and parent-based approaches are similarly effective to traditional CBT, representing an alternative rather than an improvement of the standard delivery format.[41,46,47]

Cognitive Behavioral Therapy Components for Anxiety Treatment

Several key components are consistent across CBT protocols with demonstrated efficacy. The primary CBT strategies emphasized for anxious youth typically include building a strong therapeutic alliance, psychoeducation, cognitive restructuring, and exposure.[4,25]

Therapeutic alliance refers to the rapport between the patient and the clinician. At the beginning of the treatment, this is often done by engaging in conversations about the child or adolescents' interest, their daily lives, their motivation for seeking treatment, or by playing games. These practices are extended throughout the treatment, often by setting aside a few minutes to play games or watch videos at the end of sessions.[48] The quality of the therapeutic alliance has been shown to positively affect outcomes, although this effect is modest for anxiety disorders, with meta-analytic findings estimating an effect size of 0.10 to 0.14.[49–52] There is some evidence to suggest that with younger children and children with mixed symptom presentations, the importance of the therapeutic alliance may be stronger than usual.[51,52]

Psychoeducation is the process of increasing the child or adolescents, and their caregivers, overall knowledge of the relevant anxiety disorder and its treatment. This includes discussing what the symptoms feel like, where they come from, how they work, what impact they have, how treatment will progress, and dispelling myths and misperceptions about the diagnosis. High patient engagement in the psychoeducational component of CBT has been shown to positively predict treatment response in youth.[53]

Cognitive restructuring involves teaching the child or adolescent to identify, evaluate, and modify faulty thoughts, evaluations, and beliefs that are contributing to or maintaining their symptoms.[54] The patient's level of cognitive development influences the relative utility of this component to some extent, where older youth may derive greater benefit from mastery of these skills, and the benefits may be less for children under the age of 10 or who have not yet developed meta-cognition.[55] Nevertheless, research on CBT for youth suggests that the cognitive restructuring component of treatment represents an active feature of change.[48,56]

Exposure is the main behavioral component of CBT for anxiety.[48,57,58] In CBT for children and adolescents, exposures typically follow a graded approach in which patients, with their caregivers and therapist, identify feared or anxiety-provoking situations and rank them in terms of difficulty. They begin with facing the easiest situation and gradually move up to more challenging scenarios as they progress through the treatment. Historically, the rationale for exposure was based on emotion processing theory,[59] which emphasized that the client's distress should decrease substantially during a session before moving on to a more challenging situation.[58] More recently, experimental studies have highlighted the role of inhibitory learning during the exposure process.[60,61] Within an inhibitory learning approach, the primary goal of exposure shifts from habituating to expectancy violation to strengthen extinction learning, and the fear-hierarchy is perhaps less strongly adhered to.[62,63] A recent meta-analysis of 75 studies found that for CBT with anxious youth, effect sizes were positively associated with the amount of in-session exposure.[64] When the exposure component of anxiety treatment is introduced, the rate of improvement on measures of symptom severity and global functioning accelerates.[56,65] Further, exposure to feared situations, although often initially uncomfortable and challenging for patients and therapists, has been found to enhance, rather than harm, the therapeutic alliance. This finding is consistent across various reports, whether from the child, the therapist, or the parent.[66,67]

COGNITIVE BEHAVIORAL THERAPY FOR DEPRESSION

CBT for adolescent depression has evolved through the integration of behavioral, cognitive, and social problem-solving theoretic models, each highlighting different aspects of the maintenance factors of depression.

Current Evidence

CBT has been consistently shown to be an effective treatment for child and adolescent depression, outperforming wait-list and attention-control conditions.[68,69] Key adaptations of CBT for adults were made for youth in the 1990s, focusing on psychoeducation, problem-solving, cognitive restructuring, behavioral activation, and social skills, with early studies demonstrating the efficacy of these adapted CBT programs,[70–73] and finding remission rates of 40% to 60% after treatment.[72,74]

The landmark Treatment for Adolescents with Depression Study found that a combination of fluoxetine and CBT, and fluoxetine alone, were superior to CBT alone after 12 weeks.[75] However, at the 36-week follow-up, there was no difference between treatments, with response rates of 81%, 81%, and 86% for CBT alone, fluoxetine alone, and the combined treatment, respectively.[76]

The Treatment of SSRI-Resistant Depression in Adolescents study provided evidence for the benefits of adding CBT to medication for those not responding to initial treatment, with significant improvements noted when CBT was included.[77] In contrast, the Adolescent Depression Antidepressant and Psychotherapy Trial found no added benefit of CBT when combined with fluoxetine, raising questions about the incremental effectiveness of CBT in more complex cases with higher levels of comorbidities.[78]

Considering that CBT may be more effective for mild/moderate depression as opposed to moderate/severe depression,[79] the optimal use may be as part of a combined treatment strategy, particularly in complex cases or when initial medication treatment does not lead to improvements.[78]

Cognitive Behavioral Therapy Components for Depression Treatment

Initially, behavioral models suggested that depression may stem from low levels of positive reinforcement, with affected individuals reporting fewer pleasant activities.[80–82] Stressful events and poor coping responses could then reduce positive reinforcement even further and increase negative experiences. The primary goal of behavioral treatments in CBT is to increase engagement in reinforcing activities and develop stress-coping strategies.[83]

Cognitive theories attribute depression to information processing errors that foster negative self-views and dysfunctional attitudes, leading to negative self-schemas.[84] Cognitive therapy components focus on identifying and revising these thought patterns and forming a more balanced self-schema. Cognitive therapy also addresses depressive attributional styles, rumination, and beliefs about personal competence or control.[85]

A third model, the social problem-solving theory, suggests that ineffective problem-solving skills are associated with depression. This theory advocates for a systemic approach to identifying and implementing solutions to problems.[86] Most modern CBT approaches integrate aspects from all 3 models to effectively treat youth depression.[87]

CBT sessions, whether for anxiety or depression, should have a consistent structure with standard elements like agenda setting, goal review, homework review, safety checks, session summaries, and the development of new tasks. Strategies must be taught through active patient engagement, role-playing, and experiential learning rather than passive listening. The therapist's role is to ensure the adolescent is actively participating and internalizing the skills taught during therapy sessions.[87]

In treating youth depression, establishing a strong therapeutic alliance is crucial and the relationship between the client and the therapist is promoted during the entire treatment process.[48] Psychoeducation is also important, to establish a shared understanding of the youth's depression. High patient engagement in the psychoeducational component of CBT has been shown to positively predict treatment response in youth.[53] Early in treatment goal setting, where the adolescents define what they want to improve in their lives, with the therapist breaking these into actionable steps, takes place in a collaborative effort. Mood monitoring is also taught early on to help the youth recognize the impact of CBT strategies on their feelings. Regular progress reviews are conducted throughout as they are important to reinforce self-efficacy.

The focus of treatment is on the 3 core strategies of CBT for depression. Research has demonstrated the effectiveness of each of these strategies, either as standalone treatments or as part of a comprehensive therapy.[88,89] Clinicians should focus on these strategies, while also incorporating additional techniques as required.[90] They are

1. Behavioral activation,[88] where adolescents learn that engaging in activities, particularly pleasant and social activities, can improve symptoms.[91] In practice, this often simply takes the form of helping the adolescent schedule and engage in more adaptive, preferably pleasant, daily activities, which over time improves mood and functioning.[92]
2. Cognitive restructuring, which focuses on changing negative thought patterns. As in the treatment of anxiety, this component involves teaching the adolescent to

recognize and change maladaptive thinking and appraisals[54] and has been found to be integral in CBT.[48,56,93]

3. Problem-solving, which enhances behavioral and cognitive flexibility by teaching adolescents to actively manage life challenges.[86] The therapist uses a stepwise method, incorporating emotional expression and acceptance that problems are a natural part of life.

FUTURE DIRECTIONS

Although evidence-based treatments such as CBT are clearly beneficial for youth with anxiety or depressive disorders, many affected children and adolescents do not access these treatments for various reasons.[94] Technology-based interventions have emerged as transformative tools that combine the capabilities of modern technology with traditional CBT. They may offer multiple benefits, including saving therapist time, allowing patients to work independently, decreasing the stigma of therapy, and overcoming geographic and physical barriers.[95,96] These treatments can also track progress, offer varied audiovisual instructions tailored to patients' preferences, and can be integrated into daily life using tools like smartphone apps.[97,98] Smartphone apps can also supplement clinic-based CBT by collecting data on a day-to-day basis.[99] However, high dropout rates remain a challenge, especially in unguided interventions.[100,101] Meta-analyses, primarily based on randomized controlled trials focusing on treatments for anxiety or depression, indicate the potential benefits of technology-based interventions on the mental health of children and young people, although the effectiveness can vary.[102] However, there is still a need for a more comprehensive understanding of the specific characteristics that influence their efficacy.[103–105]

The effectiveness of CBT for anxiety and depression in comparison to other evidence-based treatments, especially antidepressants remain inconclusive.[25,26,69] This could be an area of future study as well as work aiding the choice of best treatment for each patient. Future work on strengthening the effects of CBT might also include the use of predictor studies to highlight poor prognostic characteristics that might need to be specifically addressed,[106] decision-making flowcharts to tailor modular treatment components to each case,[107] a more thorough examination of change mechanisms in CBT, and the use of more objective, observational, or neuroscience-based measures,[108] and their role in predicting treatment responses.[109] Furthermore, understanding if achieving clinical remission through CBT can help anxious youth discontinue medications—as has been shown in adults with obsessive-compulsive disorder—remains uncertain.[110] These areas merit further investigation.

SUMMARY

Anxiety and depression are highly prevalent in children and adolescents and are associated with high functional impairment. Early intervention offers the best opportunity to positively impact the trajectory of depressed and anxious children. Clinician-administered instruments, as well as parent-report and youth-report questionnaires, are the most used methods to assess anxiety and depression symptoms in youth. Ideally, assessments for youth should use multiple methods and involve multiple informants. CBT for anxiety disorders in children and adolescents has a robust evidence base. CBT for depression also has strong research support, but its optimal use may be as part of a combined treatment strategy, particularly in complex cases. CBT for both anxiety and depression focuses on building a strong therapeutic alliance and incorporates psychoeducation and cognitive restructuring. In addition, anxiety treatment strongly emphasizes exposure, while depression treatment focuses on behavioral activation and problem-solving. Future directions include improving access through technology and improving effectiveness through personalization and greater understanding of mechanisms of change.

CLINICS CARE POINTS

- When assessing anxiety and depression, a multi-method multi-informant approach is recommended.

- During CBT, clinicians should ensure the establishment of a strong rapport with the child and take care to involve both the child and their parent during psychoeducation.

- Anxiety treatment should involve cognitive restructuring and strongly emphasize the exposure component, utilizing an inhibitory learning approach.

- For depression, clinicians should focus on 3 core strategies: behavioral activation, problem-solving, and cognitive restructuring, alongside additional techniques tailored to the individual's needs.

- For depression, consider CBT as part of a combined treatment strategy, especially in complex cases or when initial medication does not lead to improvements.

DISCLOSURE

O. Smárason and G. Skarphedinsson have no conflict of interest to report. Dr E.A. Storch reports receiving research funding to his institution from the REAM Foundation, United States, International OCD Foundation, United States, and National Institutes of Health, United States. He was formerly a consultant for Brainsway and Biohaven Pharmaceuticals in the past 12 months. He owns stock less than $5000 in NView. He receives book royalties from Elsevier, Wiley, Oxford, American Psychological Association, Guildford, Springer, Routledge, and Jessica Kingsley.

REFERENCES

1. Merikangas KR, He, Burstein, et al. Lifetime prevalence of mental disorders in U.S. adolescents: results from the National Comorbidity Survey Replication–Adolescent Supplement (NCS-A). J Am Acad Child Adolesc Psychiatry 2010; 49(10):980–9.
2. Beesdo K, Knappe S, Pine DS. Anxiety and anxiety disorders in children and adolescents: developmental issues and implications for DSM-V. Psychiatr Clin North Am 2009;32(3):483–524.
3. Huberty TJ. Anxiety and depression in children and adolescents: assessment, intervention, and prevention. New York, NY: Springer Science & Business Media; 2012.
4. van Beljouw IMJ, Verhaak, Cuijpers, et al. The course of untreated anxiety and depression, and determinants of poor one-year outcome: a one-year cohort study. BMC Psychiatr 2010;10(1):86.
5. Scott AJ, Bisby, Heriseanu, et al. Understanding the untreated course of anxiety disorders in treatment-seeking samples: A systematic review and meta-analysis. J Anxiety Disord 2022;89:102590.

6. Woodward LJ, Fergusson DM. Life course outcomes of young people with anxiety disorders in adolescence. J Am Acad Child Adolesc Psychiatry 2001;40(9): 1086–93.

7. Langley AK, Falk, Peris, et al. The child anxiety impact scale: examining parent- and child-reported impairment in child anxiety disorders. J Clin Child Adolesc Psychol 2014;43(4):579–91.

8. Essau CA, Conradt J, Petermann F. Course and outcome of anxiety disorders in adolescents. J Anxiety Disord 2002;16(1):67–81.

9. Kessler RC, Berglund, Demler, et al. Lifetime Prevalence and Age-of-Onset Distributions of DSM-IV Disorders in the National Comorbidity Survey Replication. Arch Gen Psychiatry 2005;62(6):593–602.

10. Cole DA, Tram, Martin, et al. Individual differences in the emergence of depressive symptoms in children and adolescents: a longitudinal investigation of parent and child reports. J Abnorm Psychol 2002;111(1):156–65.

11. Costello EJ, Mustillo, Erkanli, et al. Prevalence and development of psychiatric disorders in childhood and adolescence. Arch Gen Psychiatry 2003;60(8): 837–44.

12. Albert PR. Why is depression more prevalent in women? J Psychiatry Neurosci 2015;40(4):219–21.

13. Rao U, Chen L-A. Characteristics, correlates, and outcomes of childhood and adolescent depressive disorders. Dialogues Clin Neurosci 2009;11(1):45–62.

14. Brent DA, Perper, Moritz, et al. Psychiatric Risk Factors for Adolescent Suicide: A Case-Control Study. Journal of the American Academy of Child & Adolescent Psychiatry 1993;32(3):521–9.

15. Dunn V, Goodyer IM. Longitudinal investigation into childhood- and adolescence-onset depression: psychiatric outcome in early adulthood. Br J Psychiatry 2006;188(3):216–22.

16. Spence SH. Assessing anxiety disorders in children and adolescents. Child Adolesc Ment Health 2018;23(3):266–82.

17. Birmaher B, Khetarpal, Brent, et al. The Screen for Child Anxiety Related Emotional Disorders (SCARED): scale construction and psychometric characteristics. J Am Acad Child Adolesc Psychiatry 1997;36(4):545–53.

18. Chorpita BF, Yim, Moffitt, et al. Assessment of symptoms of DSM-IV anxiety and depression in children: a revised child anxiety and depression scale. Behav Res Ther 2000;38(8):835–55.

19. Silverman WK, Albano AM. Anxiety disorders interview schedule for DSM-IV: child Version. San Antonio, TX: The Psychologial Corporation/Graywind Publications; 1996.

20. Kaufman J, Birmaher, Brent, et al. Schedule for Affective Disorders and Schizophrenia for School-Age Children-Present and Lifetime Version (K-SADS-PL): initial reliability and validity data. J Am Acad Child Adolesc Psychiatry 1997; 36(7):980–8.

21. Easden MH, Kazantzis N. Case conceptualization research in cognitive behavior therapy: A state of the science review. J Clin Psychol 2018;74(3): 356–84.

22. Beck JS. Cognitive behavior therapy: Basics and beyond. Guilford Publications; 2020.

23. Rachman S. Psychological treatment of anxiety: the evolution of behavior therapy and cognitive behavior therapy. Annu Rev Clin Psychol 2009;5:97–119.

24. Brewin CR. Theoretical foundations of cognitive-behavior therapy for anxiety and depression. Annu Rev Psychol 1996;47(1):33–57.

25. Sigurvinsdóttir AL, Jensínudóttir KB, Baldvinsdóttir KD, et al. Effectiveness of cognitive behavioral therapy (CBT) for child and adolescent anxiety disorders across different CBT modalities and comparisons: a systematic review and meta-analysis. Nord J Psychiatry 2020;74(3):168–80.

26. Wang Z, Whiteside SPH, Sim L, et al. Comparative Effectiveness and Safety of Cognitive Behavioral Therapy and Pharmacotherapy for Childhood Anxiety Disorders: A Systematic Review and Meta-analysis. JAMA Pediatr 2017;171(11): 1049–56.

27. Rapee RM, Lyneham, Wuthrich, et al. Comparison of Stepped Care Delivery Against a Single, Empirically Validated Cognitive-Behavioral Therapy Program for Youth With Anxiety: A Randomized Clinical Trial. J Am Acad Child Adolesc Psychiatry 2017;56(10):841–8.

28. Norris LA, Kendall PC. A Close Look Into Coping Cat: Strategies Within an Empirically Supported Treatment for Anxiety in Youth. J Cogn Psychother 2020;34(1):4–20.

29. Hudson JL, Rapee, Lyneham, et al. Comparing outcomes for children with different anxiety disorders following cognitive behavioural therapy. Behav Res Ther 2015;72:30–7.

30. Walkup JT, Albano, Piacentini, et al. Cognitive behavioral therapy, sertraline, or a combination in childhood anxiety. N Engl J Med 2008;359(26):2753–66.

31. Piacentini J, Bennett, Compton, et al. 24- and 36-week outcomes for the Child/Adolescent Anxiety Multimodal Study (CAMS). J Am Acad Child Adolesc Psychiatry 2014;53(3):297–310.

32. Arnardóttir A, Skarphedinsson G. Comparative effectiveness of cognitive behavioral treatment, serotonin, and serotonin noradrenaline reuptake inhibitors for anxiety in children and adolescents: a network meta-analysis. Nord J Psychiatr 2023;77(2):118–26.

33. Comer JS, Puliafico, Aschenbrand, et al. A pilot feasibility evaluation of the CALM Program for anxiety disorders in early childhood. J Anxiety Disord 2012;26(1):40–9.

34. Comer JS, Hong, Poznanski, et al. Evidence Base Update on the Treatment of Early Childhood Anxiety and Related Problems. J Clin Child Adolesc Psychol 2019;48(1):1–15.

35. Compton SN, Peris, Almirall, et al. Predictors and moderators of treatment response in childhood anxiety disorders: results from the CAMS trial. J Consult Clin Psychol 2014;82(2):212–24.

36. Evans R, Clark DM, Leigh E. Are young people with primary social anxiety disorder less likely to recover following generic CBT compared to young people with other primary anxiety disorders? A systematic review and meta-analysis. Behav Cogn Psychother 2021;49(3):352–69.

37. Beidel DC, Turner, Sallee, et al. SET-C versus fluoxetine in the treatment of childhood social phobia. J Am Acad Child Adolesc Psychiatry 2007;46(12):1622–32.

38. Spence SH, Rapee RM. The etiology of social anxiety disorder: An evidence-based model. Behav Res Ther 2016;86:50–67.

39. Scaini S, Belotti, Ogliari, et al. A comprehensive meta-analysis of cognitive-behavioral interventions for social anxiety disorder in children and adolescents. J Anxiety Disord 2016;42:105–12.

40. Lippert MW, Pflug, Lavallee, et al. Enhanced Family Approaches for the Anxiety Disorders. In: Farrell LJ, Muris P, Ollendick TH, editors. Innovations in CBT for childhood anxiety, OCD, and PTSD: improving access and outcomes. Cambridge: Cambridge University Press; 2019. p. 182–205.

41. Lebowitz ER, Marin, Martino, et al. Parent-Based Treatment as Efficacious as Cognitive-Behavioral Therapy for Childhood Anxiety: A Randomized Noninferiority Study of Supportive Parenting for Anxious Childhood Emotions. J Am Acad Child Adolesc Psychiatry 2020;59(3):362–72.

42. Ginsburg GS, Siqueland, Masia-Warner, et al. Anxiety disorders in children: Family matters. Cognit Behav Pract 2004;11(1):28–43.

43. Rapee RM. Family factors in the development and management of anxiety disorders. Clin Child Fam Psychol Rev 2012;15(1):69–80.

44. Lebowitz ER, Omer, Hermes, et al. Parent Training for Childhood Anxiety Disorders: The SPACE Program. Cognit Behav Pract 2014;21(4):456–69.

45. Creswell C, Parkinson M, Thirlwall K, et al. Parent-led CBT for child anxiety: helping parents help their kids. New York: Guilford Publications; 2019.

46. Peris TS, Thamrin H, Rozenman MS. Family Intervention for Child and Adolescent Anxiety: A Meta-analytic Review of Therapy Targets, Techniques, and Outcomes. J Affect Disord 2021;286:282–95.

47. Thirlwall K, Cooper, Karalus, et al. Treatment of child anxiety disorders via guided parent-delivered cognitive-behavioural therapy: randomised controlled trial. Br J Psychiatry 2013;203(6):436–44.

48. Kendall PC, Ney, Maxwell, et al. Adapting CBT for youth anxiety: Flexibility, within fidelity, in different settings. Front Psychiatry 2023;14:1067047.

49. Cummings CM, Caporino, Settipani, et al. The therapeutic relationship in cognitive-behavioral therapy and pharmacotherapy for anxious youth. J Consult Clin Psychol 2013;81(5):859–64.

50. Marker CD, Comer, Abramova, et al. The reciprocal relationship between alliance and symptom improvement across the treatment of childhood anxiety. J Clin Child Adolesc Psychol 2013;42(1):22–33.

51. Bose D, Proenza, Costales, et al. Therapeutic alliance in psychosocial interventions for youth internalizing disorders: A systematic review and preliminary meta-analysis. Clin Psychol Sci Pract 2022;29(2):124–36.

52. McLeod BD. Relation of the alliance with outcomes in youth psychotherapy: A meta-analysis. Clin Psychol Rev 2011;31(4):603–16.

53. Chiappini EA, Gosch, Compton, et al. In-session involvement in anxious youth receiving CBT with/without medication. J Psychopathol Behav Assess 2020; 42(4):615–26.

54. Clark DA. Cognitive restructuring. The Wiley handbook of cognitive behavioral therapy; 2013. p. 1–22. Cognitive Restructuring.

55. Waite P, Codd J, Creswell C. Interpretation of ambiguity: Differences between children and adolescents with and without an anxiety disorder. J Affect Disord 2015;188:194–201.

56. Peris TS, Compton, Kendall, et al. Trajectories of Change in Youth Anxiety During Cognitive—Behavior Therapy. J Consult Clin Psychol 2015;83(2):239–52.

57. Higa-McMillan CK, Francis, Rith-Najarian, et al. Evidence base update: 50 years of research on treatment for child and adolescent anxiety. J Clin Child Adolesc Psychol 2016;45(2):91–113.

58. Kendall PC, Robin, Hedtke, et al. Considering CBT with anxious youth? Think exposures. Cognit Behav Pract 2005;12(1):136–48.

59. Foa, E.B., J.D. Huppert, and S.P. Cahill, Emotional processing theory: An update. 2006.

60. McGuire JF, Orr, Essoe, et al. Extinction learning in childhood anxiety disorders, obsessive compulsive disorder and post-traumatic stress disorder: implications for treatment. Expert Rev Neurother 2016;16(10):1155–74.

61. Craske MG, Kircanski, Zelikowsky, et al. Optimizing inhibitory learning during exposure therapy. Behav Res Ther 2008;46(1):5–27.
62. Craske MG, Treanor, Conway, et al. Maximizing exposure therapy: An inhibitory learning approach. Behav Res Ther 2014;58:10–23.
63. McGuire JF, Storch EA. An Inhibitory Learning Approach to Cognitive-Behavioral Therapy for Children and Adolescents. Cognit Behav Pract 2018;26(1):214–24.
64. Whiteside SP, Sim, Morrow, et al. A meta-analysis to guide the enhancement of CBT for childhood anxiety: exposure over anxiety management. Clin Child Fam Psychol Rev 2020;23(1):102–21.
65. Guzick AG, Schneider, Kendall, et al. Change during cognitive and exposure phases of cognitive–behavioral therapy for autistic youth with anxiety disorders. J Consult Clin Psychol 2022;90(9):709–14.
66. Kendall PC, Comer, Marker, et al. In-session exposure tasks and therapeutic alliance across the treatment of childhood anxiety disorders. J Consult Clin Psychol 2009;77(3):517–25.
67. Buchholz JL, Abramowitz JS. The therapeutic alliance in exposure therapy for anxiety-related disorders: A critical review. J Anxiety Disord 2020;70:102194.
68. Oud M, de Winter, Vermeulen-Smit, et al. Effectiveness of CBT for children and adolescents with depression: A systematic review and meta-regression analysis. Eur Psychiatry 2019;57:33–45.
69. Zhou X, Teng, Zhang, et al. Comparative efficacy and acceptability of antidepressants, psychotherapies, and their combination for acute treatment of children and adolescents with depressive disorder: a systematic review and network meta-analysis. Lancet Psychiatr 2020;7(7):581–601.
70. Lewinsohn PM, Clarke, Hops, et al. Cognitive-behavioral treatment for depressed adolescents. Behav Ther 1990;21(4):385–401.
71. Brent DA, Holder, Kolko, et al. A clinical psychotherapy trial for adolescent depression comparing cognitive, family, and supportive therapy. Arch Gen Psychiatry 1997;54(9):877–85.
72. Clarke GN, Rohde, Lewinsohn, et al. Cognitive-Behavioral Treatment of Adolescent Depression: Efficacy of Acute Group Treatment and Booster Sessions. Journal of the American Academy of Child & Adolescent Psychiatry 1999; 38(3):272–9.
73. McCARTY CA, Weisz JR. Effects of Psychotherapy for Depression in Children and Adolescents: What We Can (and Can't) Learn from Meta-Analysis and Component Profiling. Journal of the American Academy of Child & Adolescent Psychiatry 2007;46(7):879–86.
74. Birmaher B, Brent, Kolko, et al. Clinical Outcome After Short-term Psychotherapy for Adolescents With Major Depressive Disorder. Arch Gen Psychiatry 2000;57(1):29–36.
75. March J, Silva, Petrycki, et al. Fluoxetine, cognitive-behavioral therapy, and their combination for adolescents with depression: Treatment for Adolescents With Depression Study (TADS) randomized controlled trial. JAMA 2004;292(7): 807–20.
76. The Treatment for Adolescents With Depression Study (TADS): Long-term Effectiveness and Safety Outcomes. Arch Gen Psychiatr 2007;64(10):1132–43.
77. Brent D, Emslie, Clarke, et al. Switching to another SSRI or to venlafaxine with or without cognitive behavioral therapy for adolescents with SSRI-resistant depression: the TORDIA randomized controlled trial. JAMA 2008;299(8):901–13.
78. Goodyer I, Dubicka, Wilkinson, et al. Selective serotonin reuptake inhibitors (SSRIs) and routine specialist care with and without cognitive behaviour therapy

in adolescents with major depression: randomised controlled trial. BMJ 2007;
335(7611):142.

79. Kunas SL, Lautenbacher, Lueken, et al. Psychological Predictors of Cognitive-Behavioral Therapy Outcomes for Anxiety and Depressive Disorders in Children and Adolescents: A Systematic Review and Meta-Analysis. J Affect Disord 2021;278:614–26.

80. Lewinsohn PM, Graf M. Pleasant activities and depression. J Consult Clin Psychol 1973;41(2):261–8.

81. Segrin C. Social skills deficits associated with depression. Clin Psychol Rev 2000;20(3):379–403.

82. Sheeber L, Hops H, Davis B. Family Processes in Adolescent Depression. Clin Child Fam Psychol Rev 2001;4(1):19–35.

83. Lewinsohn, P.M. and I.H. Gotlib, Behavioral theory and treatment of depression. 1995.

84. Beck AT. Cognitive therapy of depression. Guilford press; 1979.

85. Beck AT, Alford BA. Depression: Causes and treatment. University of Pennsylvania Press; 2009.

86. Nezu AM. A problem-solving formulation of depression: A literature review and proposal of a pluralistic model. Clin Psychol Rev 1987;7(2):121–44.

87. Weersing VR, Brent DA. Cognitive Behavioral Therapy for Depression in Youth. Child Adolesc Psychiatr Clin N Am 2006;15(4):939–ix.

88. McCauley E, Gudmundsen, Schloredt, et al. The Adolescent Behavioral Activation Program: Adapting Behavioral Activation as a Treatment for Depression in Adolescence. J Clin Child Adolesc Psychol 2016;45(3):291–304.

89. Kennard BD, Clarke, Weersing, et al. Effective components of TORDIA cognitive–behavioral therapy for adolescent depression: Preliminary findings. J Consult Clin Psychol 2009;77(6):1033–41.

90. Fang H, Tu, Sheng, et al. Depression in sleep disturbance: A review on a bidirectional relationship, mechanisms and treatment. J Cell Mol Med 2019;23(4): 2324–32.

91. Kanter JW, Manos, Bowe, et al. What is behavioral activation? A review of the empirical literature. Clin Psychol Rev 2010;30(6):608–20.

92. Martin F, Oliver T. Behavioral activation for children and adolescents: a systematic review of progress and promise. Eur Child Adolesc Psychiatr 2019;28(4): 427–41.

93. Ng M.Y., DiVasto K. A., Gonzalez N.-a-r., et al., How do cognitive behavioral therapy and interpersonal psychotherapy improve youth depression? Applying meta-analytic structural equation modeling to three decades of randomized trials, Psychol Bull, 149 (9–10), 2023, 507–548.

94. Essau CA. Frequency and patterns of mental health services utilization among adolescents with anxiety and depressive disorders. Depress Anxiety 2005; 22(3):130–7.

95. Shealy KM, Davidson, Jones, et al. Delivering an evidence-based mental health treatment to underserved populations using telemedicine: The case of a trauma-affected adolescent in a rural setting. Cognit Behav Pract 2015;22(3):331–44.

96. Wolters LH, Weidle, Babiano-Espinosa, et al. Feasibility, Acceptability and Effectiveness of Enhanced Cognitive Behavioral Therapy (eCBT) for Children and Adolescents With Obsessive-Compulsive Disorder: Therapeutic Intervention and Trial Protocol. JMIR Res Protoc 2020;9(12):e24057.

97. Aspvall K, Andersson, Melin, et al. Effect of an internet-delivered stepped-care program vs in-person cognitive behavioral therapy on obsessive-compulsive

disorder symptoms in children and adolescents: a randomized clinical trial. JAMA 2021;325(18):1863–73.

98. Jones S, Wainwright, Jovanoska, et al. An exploratory randomised controlled trial of a web-based integrated bipolar parenting intervention (IBPI) for bipolar parents of young children (aged 3–10). BMC Psychiatr 2015;15:122–8.

99. Whiteside SP. Mobile device-based applications for childhood anxiety disorders. J Child Adolesc Psychopharmacol 2016;26(3):246–51.

100. Karyotaki E, Kleiboer, Smit, et al. Predictors of treatment dropout in self-guided web-based interventions for depression: an 'individual patient data' meta-analysis. Psychol Med 2015;45(13):2717–26.

101. van Ballegooijen W, Cuijpers, van Straten, et al. Adherence to Internet-based and face-to-face cognitive behavioural therapy for depression: a meta-analysis. PLoS One 2014;9(7):e100674.

102. Hollis C, Falconer, Martin, et al. Annual Research Review: Digital health interventions for children and young people with mental health problems - a systematic and meta-review. J Child Psychol Psychiatry 2017;58(4):474–503.

103. Comer JS. Introduction to the special series: Applying new technologies to extend the scope and accessibility of mental health care. Cognit Behav Pract 2015;22(3):253–7.

104. Domhardt M, Geßlein, von Rezori, et al. Internet- and mobile-based interventions for anxiety disorders: A meta-analytic review of intervention components. Depress Anxiety 2019;36(3):213–24.

105. Myers K, Comer JS. The case for telemental health for improving the accessibility and quality of children's mental health services. J Child Adolesc Psychopharmacol 2016;26(3):186–91.

106. Ng MY, Weisz JR. Annual Research Review: Building a science of personalized intervention for youth mental health. J Child Psychol Psychiatry 2016;57(3):216–36.

107. Chorpita, B.F. and J.R. Weisz, MATCH-ADTC: Modular Approach to Therapy for Children with Anxiety, Depression, Trauma, or Conduct Problems, 2009.

108. Fitzpatrick OM, Cho, Venturo-Conerly, et al. Empirically Supported Principles of Change in Youth Psychotherapy: Exploring Codability, Frequency of Use, and Meta-Analytic Findings. Clin Psychol Sci 2023;11(2):326–44.

109. Forbes EE, Olino, Ryan, et al. Reward-related brain function as a predictor of treatment response in adolescents with major depressive disorder. Cogn Affect Behav Neurosci 2010;10(1):107–18.

110. Foa EB, Simpson, Gallagher, et al. Maintenance of Wellness in Patients With Obsessive-Compulsive Disorder Who Discontinue Medication After Exposure/Response Prevention Augmentation: A Randomized Clinical Trial. JAMA Psychiatr 2022;79(3):193–200.

Southampton Adaptation Framework to Culturally Adapt Cognitive Behavior Therapy
An Update

Farooq Naeem, PhD[a],*, Peter Phiri, PhD[b], Nusrat Husain, MD[c]

KEYWORDS

- Southampton adaptation framework • Culturally adapted CBT • Culture
- Cognitive therapy

KEY POINTS

- Cognitive therapy needs to be culturally adapted for clients from nonwestern background.
- Southampton adaptation framework is the most commonly used adaptation framework that has been developed to culturally adapt CBT.
- cbt should be culturally adapted using stakeholder engagement: clients and their carers, mental health professionals and community leaders and religious and spiritual healrs
- Cultural adaptation typically focuses on awareness of cultural and religious issues, assessment of cultural issues that need to be addressed in the therapy and consideration of adjustments in therapy.

Modern CBT refers to a family of interventions combining various cognitive, behavioral, and emotion-focused techniques.[1] The cognitive therapy model has evolved over the years. While initially developed as a treatment for depression, the flexibility of the model allowed adaptations for a variety of mental health problems such as anxiety, PTSD, and psychosis.[2] Further modifications led to the development of third-wave therapies such as mindfulness-based CBT,[3] Dialectical Behavior Therapy[4] and Acceptance and Commitment Therapy.[5] It is this ability to evolve that has made CBT the most popular treatment modality across the world.

The study of psychotherapy across races, religions, and cultures, or "ethno-psychotherapy,"[6] is a relatively new discipline. This article focuses on cognitive–behavioural therapy (CBT) across cultures, which we have dubbed "ethno-CBT."[7] With the fast pace of globalization, many countries are becoming culturally, religiously, and racially

[a] Department of Psychiatry, University of Toronto, Toronto, Ontario, Canada; [b] Psychology Department, Visiting Academic, University of Southampton, Southampton, England; [c] Department of Psychiatry, University of Manchester, Manchester, England
* Corresponding author. 10 White Squirrel Way, Toronto, ON M6J 1H4.
E-mail address: farooqnaeem@yahoo.com

Psychiatr Clin N Am 47 (2024) 325–341
https://doi.org/10.1016/j.psc.2024.02.009
0193-953X/24/© 2024 Elsevier Inc. All rights reserved.

diverse; therefore, there is a drive toward improving equity in health care in most countries in the global north.[8] This implies that to be responsive to the needs of people, the health care systems must address disparities by providing equitable, culturally responsive, and effective clinical services to diverse populations. The inability to provide culturally competent health care leads to a gap in services for people from ethnic minority cultures that, in turn, leads to poor access to available services, poor outcomes, and increasing costs to society.[9] On the other hand, improving economic conditions in Asian and South American countries[10] and growing awareness of evidence-based psychological interventions have increased demand for evidence-based interventions. Unlike surgical or medical interventions, psychological therapies must consider social, cultural, political, and religious factors.

COGNITIVE BEHAVIOR THERAPY AND CULTURE

Culture is hard to define. Some authorities suggest that the material (infrastructure, and so forth) and the subjective aspects (lifestyle, attitudes, customs, and values) of the world in which a person lives together constitute a person's culture.[11] Others suggest that only the nonmaterial aspects of a person's environment constitute their culture.[12] The UNESCO (United Nations Educational, Scientific, and Cultural Organization) defines culture as "the set of distinctive spiritual, material, intellectual, and emotional features of society or a social group, and it encompasses, in addition to art and literature, lifestyles, ways of living together, value systems, traditions, and beliefs."[13] UNESCO also emphasizes cultural diversity, promotes cultural pluralism, delineates cultural diversity and asserts that it presupposes respect for human rights. This definition provides the foundation on which the cultural adaptation of evidence-based psychological interventions rests.

There is now sufficient evidence that culture can influence the process and outcomes of psychological interventions.[14,15] It has been observed that "because white males from the West developed most psychotherapy theories, they may conflict with the cultural values and beliefs of clients from non-Western backgrounds."[16] Therapists working with diverse populations have pointed out that Eastern and Western cultures differ in 4 core value dimensions: individualism–communalism, cognitivism– emotionalism, freewill–determinism and.[17] While these dichotomies might not reflect the true picture, especially because of the Westernization of the East and Easternization of the West (eg, popularity of Western fast-food chains in Asian countries and the East and South Asian food in the West representing the fast-changing cultural environments), they do indicate fundamental differences in people's attitudes toward life across the globe. It, therefore, surmises that CBT should be culturally adapted for it to be effective for persons from non-Western cultures.[18]

Most world religions originated from the East or the Middle East and still influence people's lives in these regions. The monotheistic faiths take a deterministic view of life, and these beliefs dominate most societies in the Global South. Opinions on free will and determinism significantly influence people's beliefs about the "cause and effect relationship." Accordingly, natural disasters, accidents, and physical and mental health problems are all divine manifestations. The Hindus and Buddhists believe in karma, which implies a direct relationship between cause and effect. However, there is disagreement on the question of free will among Hindu theosophy's six orthodox schools (Astika). The religions also promote the value of brotherhood and social hierarchy. Holy scriptures such as the Bible, Quran, and Vedas all promote respect for parents and the elders (Exodus 20:12, Quran 17:23). The philosophers of the East promoted these values further; for example, Confucius emphasizes the role of respect for parents and the elderly (filial piety), love for the family, social hierarchy, interpersonal harmony, and the importance of academic success on one hand and discourages self-centeredness (Individualism) on the other hand.[19]

Similarly, the Latino culture places enormous importance on the concept of "respect," and has strong religious beliefs and a deterministic view of life.[20,21] People from the Afro-Caribbean cultures have also been reported to believe in supernatural causes of physical and mental illnesses.[22] Taoism emphasizes a simple life, connection with nature and noninterference during natural events.[19] As a result, natural remedies remain popular in Asian countries for both physical and mental health problems. Respecting educated persons with a higher status in Asian cultures means a collaborative approach might not work with many Asian clients.

CULTURALLY ADAPTED COGNITIVE BEHAVIOR THERAPY (CULTURALLY ADAPT COGNITIVE BEHAVIOR THERAPY)

People with mental and emotional health difficulties have unhelpful thinking styles and beliefs about self, others, and the world.[23] The CBT therapist explores unhelpful thinking patterns and core beliefs and helps the person modify them. While cognitive errors are universal, the core beliefs and underlying assumptions vary across cultures.[24] CBT might be considered culturally incongruent in some cases; for example, a study from India reported that 82% of psychology students felt that the principles underlying cognitive therapy were in conflict with their value system and beliefs.[16] Nearly half thought it conflicted with their cultural values (46%) or religious beliefs (40%). Student participants in a similar study in Pakistan reported that CBT clashed with their family, social and, most importantly, religious values.[25] Qualitative studies to explore the views of mental health professionals in Pakistan, England, China, the Middle East, Africa, and Canada consistently reported the need to adapt CBT culturally.[19,26–30]

We have defined the cultural adaptation of CBT as "making adjustments in how therapy is delivered, through the acquisition of awareness, knowledge, and skills related to a given culture, without compromising on the theoretic underpinning of CBT."[31]

FRAMEWORKS TO CULTURALLY ADAPT COGNITIVE BEHAVIOR THERAPY

To address the cultural variations, therapists in the USA developed adaptation guidelines and frameworks for psychological interventions.[2] However, these early attempts were based on therapists' personal experience of working with ethnic minority clients, especially American blacks, Latin, and Chinese.[2] These frameworks describe issues related to the cultural adaptation of therapies. While some frameworks outline general guidance, others describe the cultural adaptation of specific demographics or therapies. In a recent literature review, we identified 18 adaptation frameworks.[2] None of the frameworks was the direct outcome of research that engaged stakeholders, and only 2 were used to adapt therapy that was tested in RCTs; 3 RCTs tested Bernal's framework,[32–34] while one tested Reniscow's framework.[35]

Types and Areas of Adaptations

A review of meta-analyses of culturally adapted psychological interventions reported that most adaptations focused on language, family, content, context, and access.[36] One literature review of culturally adapted interventions for Schizophrenia reported 9 core themes: language, concepts, and illness models, family, communication, content, cultural norms and practices, context and delivery, therapeutic alliance, and treatment goals.[37] Another literature review of culturally adapted interventions noted that "an explicit statement of culture, use of the client's preferred language, matched race or ethnicity between the client and the therapist, incorporation of cultural values and worldview into sessions, collaboration with cultural others, appropriately localized services, and relevant spirituality discussion work best.[38]

Experts in this area have emphasized the role of psychoeducation.[39,40] Psychoeducation indeed is an essential component of culturally adapted interventions since many clients from non-Western cultures might be unaware of the Western model of mental illness and even of psychological interventions.[41–44] The context of intervention is also essential, and it has been suggested that delivering interventions at home improves engagement and therapy outcomes,[39] possibly to avoid the stigma associated with attending a mental health center. The intervention is also likely to be more effective if the therapist and the client speak the same language.[38,45]

Working with families is an essential aspect of cultural adaptation since decisions are made as a family in some non-western cultures.[6,43] Interventions are more effective, and patient outcomes improve when patients attend with family members rather than alone.[37] Similarly, therapeutic alliance has been reported to improve if a family member is involved in therapy.[43,46] Family members can also work as co-therapists, helping clients with homework and ensuring compliance and attendance in therapy sessions.[6] It is, therefore, a common practice to involve families in adapted interventions.[37]

EVIDENCE FOR CULTURALLY ADAPTED INTERVENTIONS

Interventions adapted for a specific cultural group are four times more likely to be effective than interventions adapted for multiple groups.[38] A review of 12 meta-analyses reported that the majority of meta-analyses of culturally adapted found a moderate to large effect for culturally adapted interventions.[36] Of these 12 meta-analyses, most included studies that addressed various problems, processes, and populations. One review focused on Schizophrenia,[47] while 4 focused on depressive symptoms.[39,40,48,49] One review focused on Latinos,[45] while the rest included studies of different ethnic and cultural groups. Two reviews focused on children[50,51] and one on women.[40] Only one review compared adapted versus unadapted interventions.[52] Only 2 reviews systematically described the nature and process of cultural adaptation used in trials.[47,49] Meta-analyses report many limitations of the included studies.

SOUTHAMPTON ADAPTATION FRAMEWORK FOR CULTURALLY ADAPTING COGNITIVE BEHAVIOR THERAPY

The Southampton Adaptation Framework is the first framework explicitly developed to culturally adapt CBT.[53] It was developed through qualitative studies to engage stakeholders: patients, carers, lay persons, community leaders, faith and religious leaders, and psychologists. This framework has been used to adapt CBT for depression and anxiety in Saudi Arabia,[27] Kenya[54] and Morocco,[28] and for psychosis in Pakistan,[55] China[19] and England,[56] it has also been used in Canada to adapt DBT for clients with learning disability[57] and depression among the South Asians.[30,43,58] Please see **Table 1** for details of studies that used a culturally adapted intervention using the Southampton adaptation framework.

Development of Southampton Adaptation Framework for Culturally Adapting Cognitive Behavior Therapy

We started with a thorough literature review and meetings with field experts. A series of qualitative studies substantiated by the ethnographic approach were conducted. The information thus obtained was analyzed, and guidelines were developed to guide the development of a culturally adapted CBT manual. Culturally adapted CBT was evaluated for feasibility, acceptability, and effectiveness in a pilot study.[59]

Table 1
Characteristics of studies that used a culturally adapted intervention using the Southampton Adaptation Framework

	Author, Year	Study Type	Treatment Conditions	Problem Areas	Sample Size	Primary Outcome	Secondary Outcome	Recruitment	Population	Assessments
1	Naeem et al,[1] 2014	RCT	Treatment (CaCBT-based Guided Self-help, Control (TAU)	Depression, anxiety	Treatment (n = 94) Control (n = 89)	Depression Anxiety	Somatic complaints, Disability, Quality of life	Three University Psychiatry Departments, Pakistan	18–65 y, both genders, at least 5 y of schooling	Baseline, 12 wk
2	Butt et al,[2] 2020	RCT, Pilot	Treatment (Culturally adapted DBT), Control (TAU)	Borderline Personality Disorder	Treatment (n = 34) Control (n = 34)	Borderline Personality Traits	None	Psychiatric outpatient departments, Lahore, Pakistan	18–65 y, both genders	Baseline, 16, 32, 48 wk
3	Habib et al.,[3] 2014	RCT, Pilot	Treatment (CaCBT for psychosis), Control (TAU)	Schizophrenia	Treatment (n = 21) Control (n = 21)	Positive symptoms	Negative symptoms, delusions, hallucinations, insight	Inpatient psychiatry units of three hospitals Lahore, Pakistan	18–65 y, both genders	Baseline, 24 wk
4	Husain, O, et al,[4] 2021	RCT, Pilot	Treatment (Culturally adapted family intervention-CuLFI) Control arm (TAU)	Schizophrenia	Treatment (n = 14) Control (n = 14)	Feasibility, acceptability	Positive symptoms, negative symptoms	Psychiatric outpatient departments, three hospitals, Karachi, Pakistan	Families living with patients with Schizophrenia	Baseline, 24 wk
5	Husain, N, et al,[5] 2021	Cluster randomized controlled trial	Treatment (LTP plus), Control (TAU)	Maternal depression	Treatment (n = 402) Control (n = 372)	Maternal depression	Depression, anxiety, quality of life, social support, parenting competence	Rural areas, Sindh, Pakistan	Mothers aged 18–44 y with children aged 0–30 month old	Baseline, 12 and 24 wk

(continued on next page)

Table 1
(continued)

Author, Year	Study Type	Treatment Conditions	Problem Areas	Sample Size	Primary Outcome	Secondary Outcome	Recruitment	Population	Assessments
6 Husain, N, et al,[6] 2018	RCT	Treatment (Culturally adapted manual-assisted problem-solving training (C-MAP), Control (TAU)	Suicidal ideation	Treatment (n = 108) Control (n = 113)	Suicidal ideation	Hopelessness, depression, coping resources, healthcare utilisation.	Medical units of three university hospitals in Pakistan	Individuals aged 16–64 y	Baseline, 12 wk
7 Jones et al,[7] 2021	RCT, Pilot	Treatment (Dialectical behavior therapy adapted for Intellectual disability), Control (TAU)	Emotional dysregulation in persons with Intellectual disability	Treatment (n = 10) Control (n = 10)	Feasibility, acceptability	Emotional regulation, anger and mental health	Residential, group homes, supported independent living, Kingston, Canada	18–65 y, both genders	Baseline, 12 wk
8 Latif et al,[8] 2021	RCT, Pilot	Treatment (*Online* culturally adapted CBT-based guided self-help (CaCBT-GSH) Control (TAU)	Depression, anxiety	Treatment (n = 20), Control (n = 19)	Feasibility, acceptability	Depression, Anxiety	Adults aged 18–65 y, Karachi, Pakistan	Family physicians, General medical outpatient clinics	Baseline, 12 wk
9 Naeem et al,[9] 2015	RCT	Treatment (brief Culturally adapted CBT (CaCBT) for depression Control (TAU)	Depression	Treatment (n = 69) Control (n = 68)	Depression	Anxiety, somatic complaints, Disability	Three University Psychiatry Departments, Pakistan	Individuals aged 18–64 y	Baseline, 12 wk, 36 wk

Study	Design	Arms	Condition	Sample size	Primary outcome	Secondary outcomes	Setting	Population	Assessment
10 Husain, N, et al,[10] 2022	RCT	Treatment (Culturally Adapted Manual Assisted Problem-Solving Training (CMAP) Control (TAU)	Self-harm	Treatment (n = 440) Control (n = 461)	Self-harm	Suicidal ideation, hopelessness, quality of life	Primary care clinics, emergency and medical units, Pakistan	Adults aged 18 and above	Baseline, 12 wk, 24 wk, 48 wk
11 Aslam et al,[11] 2015	Pilot Study	Treatment (CaCBT for OCD)	OCD	Treatment (n = 21)	Obsessional thoughts and compulsions	Anxiety, depression, disability	18–65 year old individual, Lahore, Pakistan	Outpatients with OCD	Baseline, 16 wk
12 Husain, O, et al,[12] 2017	RCT, Pilot	Treatment (CaCBT for psychosis) Control (TAU)	Schizophrenia	Treatment (n = 18) Control (n = 18)	Feasibility	Positive symptoms, negative symptoms	Individuals aged 18–65 y, Karachi, Pakistan	Outpatient psychiatric services	Baseline, 12 wk, 24 wk
13 Husain, I, et al,[13] 2017	RCT, Pilot	Treatment (Culturally adapted psychoeducation (CaPE), Control (TAU)	Bipolar affective disorder	Treatment arm (n = 16) Control (n = 11)	Feasibility, acceptability	Knowledge and attitudes, adherence to medication, mood symptoms, quality of life	Individuals aged 18–65 y, Karachi, Pakistan	age 18–65 y adults	Baseline, 12 wk
14 Notiar et,[14] 2021	RCT, Pilot	Treatment [LTP plus (LTP plus CaCBT)], Control (TAU)	Maternal depression	Treatment (n = 17)	Feasibility, acceptability	Maternal depression, quality of life	Community in one district, Kenya	Women, 18–45 y with children up to 36 mo	Baseline, 12 wk
15 Naeem et al,[15] 2015	RCT	Treatment (Brief CaCBT for psychosis), Control (TAU)	Schizophrenia	Treatment (n = 59) Control (n = 49)	Positive symptoms	Negative symptoms, disability	Hospital outpatients, Lahore, Pakistan	18–65 y individuals	Baseline, 16 wk
16 Naeem et al,[16] 2010	RCT, Pilot	Treatment (CaCBT for depression) Control (TAU)	Depression	Treatment (n = 17) Control (n = 17)	Depression	Anxiety and somatic symptoms	Primary care, Lahore, Pakistan	Primary care clinics	Baseline, 12 wk

(continued on next page)

Table 1
(continued)

Author, Year	Study Type	Treatment Conditions	Problem Areas	Sample Size	Primary Outcome	Secondary Outcome	Recruitment	Population	Assessments
17 Latif et al,[17] 2021	RCT, Pilot	Treatment (CaCBT-based GSH for PTSD), Control (TAU)	PTSD	Treatment (n = 25) Control (n = 25)	Feasibility and acceptability	PTSD, depression, anxiety, disability	18–65 year old female, Karachi, Pakistan	Shelter homes	Baseline, 12 wk
18 Rathod, et al,[18] 2013	RCT, Pilot	Treatment (CaCBT for Psychosis), Control (TAU)	Schizophrenia	Treatment (n = 16) Control (n = 17)	Psychopathology	Positive symptoms, hallucinations, insight, satisfaction	18–65 year old, both genders, South Asians and Afro-Caribbeans, England	Outpatient psychiatric services	Baseline, 24 wk, 48 wk
19 Naeem et al,[19] 2023	RCT	Treatment (CaCBT), Control (Standard CBT)	Depression	Treatment (n = 75) Control (n = 71)	Feasibility, acceptability	Depression, anxiety, disability, therapeutic alliance	18–65 year old, South Asian, Canada		
20 Amin et al,[20] 2020	RCT	Treatment (CaCBT-based GSH), Control (TAU)	Self-esteem, social anxiety	Treatment (n = 38) Control (n = 38)	Self-esteem	Social anxiety, Stress	13–16 y aged adolescents, Multan, Pakistan	Schools	Baseline, 8 wk
21 Husain, N, et al,[21] 2017	RCT	Treatment (LTP Plus), Control (TAU)	Maternal depression	Treatment (n = 124) Control (n = 123)	Maternal depression	Stress in parent-child relations, self-esteem, social support, disability	Primary care clinics, Sindh, Pakistan	Women aged 18–35 y	Baseline, 12 wk
22 Husain, N, et al,[22] 2021	RCT	Treatment (Learning through Play + Thinking Healthy Program- LTP Plus), Control (TAU)	Maternal Depression	Treatment (n = 54) Control (n = 53)	Maternal Depression	Child health outcomes	Pediatric departments of two tertiary care hospitals in Pakistan	18–44-y, mothers with children 0–30 month old	Baseline, 12 wk, 24 wk

The methods of development have been described in detail elsewhere.[41] In short, qualitative interviews were used to gather information from the stakeholders,[1] patients with depression and anxiety were interviewed to understand their cultural orientation, including their beliefs about illness, its causes and the treatment, especially nonmedical treatments including the patient's experience of any nonpharmacological help received,[2] carers make treatment decisions for the patients and therefore were interviewed to explore their views about the problem, its causes and treatment, as well as their beliefs about help-seeking and any nonpharmacological treatment,[3] mental health professionals were interviewed to identify barriers and difficulties they face when helping clients from under study population, they were also asked questions to identify techniques that were easy to use and were helpful as well as techniques that or were not so helpful and required modifications,[4] university students were engaged in focus groups to explore their views about compatibility of CBT with their personal, social and religious values,[25] finally[4] further information was gathered from lay persons, community leaders and spiritual and religious leaders through informal meetings and incorporated in guidelines as field notes. A name-the-title technique was used to find equivalent terminology rather than literal translations.[60]

Our initial work included 3 studies. The Pakistani project included open-ended interviews with clinical psychologists (n = 5),[26] depressed patients (n = 9),[44] focus groups with University students (n = 34)[25] and field observations that included informal conversations with lay persons, as well as community leaders and religious and spiritual scholars. In the UK project, in-depth, face-to-face, semi-structured interviews and focus group interviews were conducted with psychotic patients (n = 15), lay members from the respective communities (n = 52), CBT therapists (n = 22), and experienced health professionals working with service users from these groups (n = 25).[29] Findings from these studies guided the adaptation of therapy manuals tested in pilot RCTs for feasibility, acceptability, and effectiveness.[59,61] In order to reduce the cost, semi-structured interviews were developed, which were used to adapt (using semi-structured interviews with 33 patients, 30 caretakers, and 29 mental health professionals)[55] and test CBT for psychosis in Pakistan.[62–64]

An overview of the process of adaptation.

In short, the development process of culturally adapted CBT comprises the following steps.

Stage 1: Review previous literature and discuss with field experts to gather initial information that will inform the adaptation process.

Stage 2: Use qualitative methods to gather information from patients and their carers to understand their views about the illness and its treatment from the therapists/mental health practitioners.

Stage 3: Formal or informal conversations with the laypersons to explore their opinion on the compatibility of CBT with their cultural or religious values.

Stage 4: Formal or informal conversations with faith healers and religious leaders to understand their perspectives on mental illness and its treatment.

Stage 5: Formal or informal conversations with health leaders and the service managers concerning their experiences and views about a particular problem and to get an idea of the successful implementation potential of the adapted intervention.

Stage 6: Translation and adaptation of the therapy manual. The therapy manual does not need to be translated if the therapists are bilingual. However, handouts and therapy material must still be adapted and translated. Most importantly, terminology should be culturally adapted.

Stage 7: Field test the adapted CBT manual's feasibility, acceptability, and effectiveness using a pilot design.

Stage 8: Further refinement of the guidelines based on a feasibility trial if required.

Stage 9: Testing the adapted therapy manual in a fully powered RCT for effectiveness.

Components of Southampton Adaptation Framework

The framework has evolved because of information from the qualitative studies conducted in different countries over the years. The framework consists of 3 major areas (the triple-A principle) of concern[1]: awareness and preparation,[2] assessment and engagement, and[3] adjustments in therapy. **Table 1** provides details of SAF-CBT components.

Culture, religion, and spirituality remain essential components of people's lives in Eastern cultures and, therefore, require full attention and exploration in this context. Culture and religion influence the cause-effect relationship.[43] People use a bio-psycho-socio-spiritual system model of illness.[41,42] For example, the cause of a mishap might be described as an "evil eye" or even "God's will." People are also likely to use religious coping strategies when dealing with distress.[65] An understanding of pathways to care and help-seeking behaviors is essential. It may be crucial for therapists to acknowledge that their clients will attend therapy and see a faith healer, an herbalist, or a magician. Involving faith healers, religious leaders, or community elders might help.[43]

Language needs to be adapted since literal translations do not work. Similarly, the involvement of family members or carers needs to be studied. The therapist should carefully assess family participation and consider both the pros and cons, everyday stressors, guilt, and stigma of mental illness in the household. Standard CBT is heavily dependent on reading and writing skills. However, this might be difficult due to low literacy rates and a reduced interest in writing in the global south. Audio tapes, diaries, beads, and counters have overcome this barrier.[6]

Clients' knowledge of and beliefs about the health system, available treatments, and the treatment providers play a significant role in their engagement with the therapist. They should be a major part of the assessment. Dysfunctional beliefs vary from culture to culture.[24,66] Beliefs related to dependence on others, the need to please other people, the need to submit to the demands of loved ones, and sacrificing one's needs for family are relatively common in non-western populations. Patients' beliefs about the illness and its treatment can be explored using structured assessment tools such as the Short Explanatory Model Interview (SEMI).[67] The Asian Cultural Identity Schedule[65] or Vancouver Index of Acculturation (VIA)[68] can be used to assess a person's cultural identity and the level of acculturation. Finally, the Dysfunctional Attitude Scale (DAS)[69] can be used with family members or community members to see whether some of the supposedly dysfunctional beliefs are acceptable within this community.

The significant barrier in providing therapy to persons from non-western cultures is the "engagement and therapeutic alliance."[70] In this regard, "culturally adapted CBT can be seen as a set of strategies to engage a client from a different cultural background." Clients from Asian backgrounds expect immediate relief; therefore, the first few sessions are critical.[42] Therapists should focus on symptom management to increase the client's confidence in the therapist's abilities. Attention to nonverbal cues can help therapists since clients might be reluctant to show disagreement or displeasure. Use of a personal touch, for example, "Oh, my mother lives in the same city where you live," examples from past successful treatments of similar problems rather than research trials, and involving family can all help improve engagement.[43]

CBT techniques require only minor adjustments.[46] Many clients from non-western cultures find it difficult to recognize and separate thoughts and emotions, possibly due to a strong "holist" position and a lack of mind-body dualism.[71] Third-wave therapies can be helpful if education on thoughts and emotions does not help. Therapists should start with somatic symptoms and behaviors.[42] Behavioral techniques such as behavioral activation, experiments, and problem-solving do not require changes. Socratic dialogue is difficult in this group and might even lead to doubts about therapists' competence. Clients expect answers from the healer and not questions. The experienced healers from these cultures use stories and images to convey their message. Understanding idioms of distress in the client's language might help. Finally, structural changes might be required, such as delivering therapy outside of the mental health care system to avoid clients feeling stigmatized (**Table 2**).

Table 2	
components of Southampton adaptation framework	
Major Areas	**Minor Areas**
Awareness of culture and religion	1. Cause and effect model of mental illness used by the population in focus (Bio-Psycho-Socio-Spiritual Model)
	2. Language and terminology (use the "name the title" technique)
	3. Communication styles, idioms of distress and personal boundaries
	4. Family and caregivers' involvement
	5. Considerations of culture-related gender and sex issues
	6. Pathways to care (traditional healers, faith healers, religious leaders, elders).
	7. Coping strategies and cultural strengths- religion, spirituality, cultural practices
	8. Health system related issues for future implementation (awareness of cognitive therapy, number of therapists, resources, distance from the treatment facility)
Assessment and engagement	1. Self-awareness in therapists about their own beliefs toward the culture of the client
	2. Common presenting complaints and concerns
	3. Assessment of acculturation and immigration status
	4. Racism and racial or other trauma and their impact on client's mental health
	5. Stigma, shame and guilt within the family and the culture
	6. Assessment of barriers to seeking therapy, engagement, application of techniques
	7. Awareness of illness, its causes, and its treatment among the members of a given culture
	8. Beliefs about illness, its causes, and its treatment among the members of a given culture
Adjustments in therapy	1. Culturally acceptable patient-therapist relationship for example, attitude toward healers
	2. Psychoeducation on symptoms, therapy and aspects of therapy, such as thoughts in a culturally acceptable manner
	3. Cultural variations in dysfunctional beliefs and content of cognitive errors
	4. Acceptable therapy settings and style
	5. Adjustments or modifications in therapy settings
	6. Use of culturally favorable communication strategies such as stories or images
	7. Knowledge and understanding of barriers in therapy, such as language, home work, and so forth
	8. Adjustments in therapy techniques

IMPLICATIONS AND FUTURE DIRECTIONS

There are wider variations and subcultures in every group of people. Racial tensions, as well as experiences related to migration and political and social systems in the host culture, should be taken into consideration. There might be wide variations, regardless of the generation, requiring an assessment of acculturation.

Cultural adaptation of psychological interventions is an emerging field; therefore, further research is needed, especially on fidelity to the principles of cultural adaptations. There is also a need for universally accepted guidelines for cultural adaptation. Most RCTs of culturally adapted therapy do not give the details of adaptation. Research is also needed to compare adapted CBT versus standard CBT and its cost-effectiveness. Implementation of culturally adapted CBT remains a significant gap in health care systems. One major gap in adaptation frameworks is the lack of stakeholder involvement during the formulation processes, as most adaptation frameworks describe the therapist's personal experience. There is no agreement on components of cultural adaptation that work; therefore, there is a need for a universally accepted framework that would ideally be supported by the International Associations for CBT to ensure global agreement. Finally, there is a need for a high-quality meta-analysis, as the current literature is almost 10 years old and consists of various psychosocial therapies from a wide range of theoretic backgrounds.

CLINICS CARE POINTS

- This article emphasizes the reasons for culturally adapted psychotherapies, especially CBT, to help individuals of minority ethnic backgrounds
- The major barriers in providing therapy for clients from a non-western background is the engagement of these clients. This can be overcome by being aware of their culture and religion and by taking into consideration cultural factors during the assessment.
- CBT can be delivered to clients from minority ethnic background without major changes in therapy techniques

DISCLOSURE

The authors declare no conflict of interest.

REFERENCES

1. Hofmann SG, Asnaani A, Vonk IJJ, et al. The efficacy of cognitive behavioral therapy: a review of meta-analyses. Cognit Ther Res 2012;36(5):427–40.
2. Naeem F, Sajid S, Naz S, et al. Culturally adapted CBT – the evolution of psychotherapy adaptation frameworks and evidence. Cognit Behav Ther 2023; 16:e10.
3. Sipe WEB, Eisendrath SJ. Mindfulness-based cognitive therapy: theory and practice. Can J Psychiatry Rev Can Psychiatr 2012;57(2):63–9.
4. Panos PT, Jackson JW, Hasan O, et al. Meta-analysis and systematic review assessing the efficacy of dialectical behavior therapy (DBT). Res Soc Work Pract 2014;24(2):213–23.

5. Ciarrochi J, Bailey A. A CBT-practitioner's guide to ACT: how to bridge the gap between cognitive behavioral therapy and acceptance and commitment therapy. New Harbinger Publications; 2008. p. 224.

6. Naeem F, Phiri P, Rathod S, et al. Cultural adaptation of cognitive–behavioural therapy. BJPsych Adv 2019;25(6):387–95.

7. Naeem F. Chapter 4 - Ethno-cognitive behavioral therapy and ethnopsychotherapy: A new narrative. In: Martin CR, Patel VB, Preedy VR, editors. Handbook of cognitive behavioral therapy by disorder [Internet]. Academic Press; 2023 [cited 2023 Nov 25]. p. 31–41. Available at: https://www.sciencedirect.com/science/article/pii/B9780323857260000181.

8. Culyer AJ, Wagstaff A. Equity and equality in health and health care. J Health Econ 1993 Dec;12(4):431–57.

9. Kirmayer LJ. Rethinking cultural competence. Transcult Psychiatr 2012 Apr 1; 49(2):149–64.

10. United Nations. Development Policy & Analysis Division | Dept of Economic & Social Affairs | United Nations. 2018 [cited 2018 Sep 15]. January 2018 Briefing on the World Economic Situation And Prospects. Available at: https://www.un.org/development/desa/dpad/publication/world-economic-situation-and-prospects-january-2018-briefing-no-110/.

11. Triandis HC, Brislin RW. Cross-cultural psychology. Am Psychol 1984;39(9):1006–16.

12. Fernando S. Mental health, race and culture. Third Edition. Third edition. Basingstoke, Hampshire ; New York, NY: Red Globe Press; 2010. p. 232.

13. UNESCO. UNESCO universal declaration on cultural diversity [Internet]. 2001. Available at: http://portal.unesco.org/en/ev.php-URL_ID=13649&URL_DO=DO_TOPIC&URL_SECTION=-471.html. [Accessed 30 March 2019].

14. Sue S, Zane N, Nagayama Hall GC, et al. The Case for Cultural Competency in Psychotherapeutic Interventions. Annu Rev Psychol 2009;60:525–48.

15. Bhui K. Culture and complex interventions: lessons for evidence, policy and practice. Br J Psychiatry 2010;197(3):172–3.

16. Scorzelli JF, Reinke-Scorzelli M. Cultural Sensitivity and Cognitive Therapy in India. Counsel Psychol 1994;22(4):603–10.

17. Laungani P. Asian perspectives in counselling and psychotherapy [Internet]. Available at:. New York: Psychology Press; 2004. https://doi.org/10.4324/9780203697085.

18. Hays PA, Iwamasa GY, editors. Culturally responsive cognitive-behavioral therapy: assessment, practice, and supervision. Washington, DC, US: American Psychological Association; 2006. p. 307, xiii.

19. Li W, Zhang L, Luo X, et al. A qualitative study to explore views of patients', carers' and mental health professionals' to inform cultural adaptation of CBT for psychosis (CBTp) in China. Available at: BMC Psychiatr 2017 [Internet]. https://www.ncbi.nlm.nih.gov/pmc/articles/PMC5385068/. [Accessed 19 March 2021].

20. Tamis-LeMonda CS, Caughy MO, Rojas R, et al. Culture, parenting, and language: Respeto in Latine mother–child interactions. Soc Dev 2020;29(3):689–712.

21. Fierros M, Smith C. The Relevance of Hispanic Culture to the Treatment of a Patient with Posttraumatic Stress Disorder (PTSD). Psychiatry Edgmont 2006;3(10):49–56.

22. Whitley R, Kirmayer LJ, Groleau D. Understanding immigrants' reluctance to use mental health services: a qualitative study from Montreal. Can J Psychiatry Rev Can Psychiatr 2006;51(4):205–9.

23. Beck AT, Emery G. Cognitive therapy of depression. 1St Edition. The Guilford Press; 1979. p. 425.
24. Sahin NH, Sahin N. How dysfunctional are the dysfunctional attitudes in another culture? Br J Med Psychol 1992;65(Pt 1):17–26.
25. Naeem F, Gobbi M, Ayub M, et al. University students' views about compatibility of cognitive behaviour therapy (CBT) with their personal, social and religious values (a study from Pakistan). Ment Health Relig Cult 2009;12(8): 847–55.
26. Naeem F, Gobbi M, Ayub M, et al. Psychologists experience of cognitive behaviour therapy in a developing country: a qualitative study from Pakistan. Int J Ment Health Syst 2010;4(2).
27. Algahtani HMS, Almulhim A, AlNajjar FA, Ali MK, Irfan M, Ayub M, et al. Cultural adaptation of cognitive behavioural therapy (CBT) for patients with depression and anxiety in Saudi Arabia and Bahrain: a qualitative study exploring views of patients, carers, and mental health professionals. Cogn Behav Ther (Internet). 2019 ed (cited 2020 Oct 4);12. Available at: https://www.cambridge.org/core/journals/the-cognitive-behaviour-therapist/article/cultural-adaptation-of-cognitive-behavioural-therapy-cbt-for-patients-with-depression-and-anxiety-in-saudi-arabia-and-bahrain-a-qualitative-study-exploring-views-of-patients-carers-and-mental-health-professionals/9A3F03C81FB18060A94237709D06D4D1/core-reader.
28. Rhermoul FZE, Naeem F, Kingdon D, et al. A qualitative study to explore views of patients, carers and mental health professionals' views on depression in Moroccan women. Int J Cult Ment Health 2017;0(0):1–16.
29. Rathod S, Kingdon D, Phiri P, et al. Developing culturally sensitive cognitive behaviour therapy for psychosis for ethnic minority patients by exploration and incorporation of service users' and health professionals' views and opinions. Behav Cognit Psychother 2010;38(5):511–33.
30. Naeem F, Khan N, Sohani N, et al. Culturally Adapted Cognitive Behaviour Therapy (CaCBT) to Improve Community Mental Health Services for Canadians of South Asian Origin: A Qualitative Study. Can J Psychiatr 2023. 07067437231178958.
31. Naeem F. Adaptation of cognitive behaviour therapy for depression in Pakistan. Lap Lambert Academic Publishing GmbH KG; 2012. p. 212.
32. Nicolas G, Arntz DL, Hirsch B, et al. Cultural adaptation of a group treatment for Haitian American adolescents. Prof Psychol Res Pract 2009;40(4):378–84.
33. Parra-Cardona JR, Bybee D, Sullivan CM, et al. Examining the impact of differential cultural adaptation with Latina/o immigrants exposed to adapted parent training interventions. J Consult Clin Psychol 2017;85(1):58–71.
34. Rosselló J, Bernal G, Rivera-Medina C. Individual and group CBT and IPT for Puerto Rican adolescents with depressive symptoms. Cult Divers Ethnic Minor Psychol 2008;14(3):234–45.
35. Pallan M, Griffin T, Hurley KL, et al. Cultural adaptation of an existing children's weight management programme: the CHANGE intervention and feasibility RCT. NIHR Journals Library 2019;23(33):1–166.
36. Rathod S, Gega L, Degnan A, et al. The current status of culturally adapted mental health interventions: a practice-focused review of meta-analyses. Neuropsychiatric Dis Treat 2018;14:165–78.
37. Degnan A, Baker S, Edge D, et al. The nature and efficacy of culturally-adapted psychosocial interventions for Schizophrenia: a systematic review and meta-analysis. Psychol Med 2018;48(5):714–27.

38. Griner D, Smith TB. Culturally adapted mental health intervention: A meta-analytic review. Psychother Theory Res Pract Train 2006;43(4):531–48.
39. Rojas-García A, Ruiz-Perez I, Rodríguez-Barranco M, et al. Healthcare interventions for depression in low socioeconomic status populations: A systematic review and meta-analysis. Clin Psychol Rev 2015;38:65–78.
40. Rojas-García A, Ruíz-Pérez I, Gonçalves DC, et al. Healthcare Interventions for Perinatal Depression in Socially Disadvantaged Women: A Systematic Review and Meta-Analysis. Clin Psychol Sci Pract 2014;21(4):363–84.
41. Naeem F, Phiri P, Munshi T, et al. Using cognitive behaviour therapy with South Asian Muslims: Findings from the culturally sensitive CBT project. Int Rev Psychiatry Abingdon Engl 2015;27(3):233–46.
42. Naeem F, Ayub M, McGuire N, David K. Culturally adapted CBT (CaCBT) for depression: Therapy manual for South Asian Muslims, . Therapists. Kindle Edition. Lahore, Pakistan: Pakistan Association of Cognitive; 2013. ISBN: 9789699920004.
43. Naeem F, Vardi G, Rao S. Culturally Adapted Cognitive Behavioural Therapy (CaCBT) for Canadians of South Asian Origin Internet. Center for Addiction and Mental Health; 2023. Available at: https://www.camh.ca/en/science-and-research/institutes-and-centres/institute-for-mental-health-policy-research/sharing-our-knowledge/culturally-adapted-cognitive-behavioural-therapy#resources.
44. Naeem F, Ayub M, Kingdon D, et al. Views of Depressed Patients in Pakistan Concerning Their Illness, Its Causes, and Treatments. Qual Health Res Internet 2012. Available at. http://qhr.sagepub.com/content/early/2012/06/15/1049732312450212. [Accessed 28 June 2012].
45. Sutton C. Culturally adapted interventions for Latinos: A meta-analysis. Sch Grad Psychol (Internet) 2015. Available at: http://commons.pacificu.edu/spp/1134.
46. Naeem F, Phiri P, Nasar A, Munshi T, Ayub M, Rathod S. An evidence-based framework for cultural adaptation of Cognitive Behaviour Therapy: Process, methodology and foci of adaptation. Psychol Med 2018;48(5):714 27, 2016;10.
47. Degnan A, Baker S, Edge D, et al. The nature and efficacy of culturally-adapted psychosocial interventions for Schizophrenia: a systematic review and meta-analysis. 2016. Psychol Med 2018;48(5):714–27.
48. van Loon A, van Schaik A, Dekker J, et al. Bridging the gap for ethnic minority adult outpatients with depression and anxiety disorders by culturally adapted treatments. J Affect Disord 2013;147(1–3):9–16.
49. Chowdhary N, Jotheeswaran AT, Nadkarni A, et al. The methods and outcomes of cultural adaptations of psychological treatments for depressive disorders: a systematic review. Psychol Med 2014;44(06):1131–46.
50. Huey S Jr, Polo AJ. Evidence-Based Psychosocial Treatments for Ethnic Minority Youth. J Clin Child Adolesc Psychol 2008;37(1):262–301.
51. Hodge DR, PhD KFJ, PhD MGV. Culturally Sensitive Interventions and Health and Behavioral Health Youth Outcomes: A Meta-Analytic Review. Soc Work Health Care 2010;49(5):401–23.
52. Benish SG, |Quintana. Culturally Adapted Psychotherapy and the Legitimacy of Myth: A Direct-Comparison Meta-Analysis. J Counsel Psychol 2011;58(3):279–89.
53. Naeem F, Ayub M, Gobbi M, Kingdon D. Journal of Pakistan Psychiatric Society. 2009 (cited 2012 Jun 10). Development of Southampton Adaptation Framework for CBT (SAF-CBT) : a framework for adaptation of CBT in non-western culture. Available at: http://www.pakmedinet.com/15940.

54. Notiar A, Jidong DE, Hawa F, et al. Treatment of maternal depression in low-in-come women: A feasibility study from Kilifi, Kenya. Available at: Int J Clin Pract 2021;75(12)   [Internet].   https://onlinelibrary.wiley.com/doi/10.1111/ijcp.14862. [Accessed 13 February 2022].

55. Naeem F, Habib N, Gul M, et al. A Qualitative Study to Explore Patients', Carers' and Health Professionals' Views to Culturally Adapt CBT for Psychosis (CBTp) in Pakistan. Behav Cognit Psychother 2014;1–13.

56. Rathod S, Phiri P, Naeem F. An evidence-based framework to culturally adapt cognitive behaviour therapy. Cogn Behav Ther (Internet). 2019 ed (cited 2019 Feb 9);12. Available at: https://www.cambridge.org/core/journals/the-cognitive-behaviour-therapist/article/an-evidencebased-framework-to-culturally-adapt-cognitive-behaviour-therapy/92E62D2508871E032F24D282A018FF72.

57. McQueen M, Blinkhorn A, Broad A, et al. Development of a cognitive behavioural therapy-based guided self-help intervention for adults with intellectual disability. J Appl Res Intellect Disabil 2018;31(5):885–96.

58. Naeem F, Tuck A, Mutta B, et al. Protocol for a multi-phase, mixed methods study to develop and evaluate culturally adapted CBT to improve community mental health services for Canadians of south Asian origin. Trials 2021; 22(1):600.

59. Naeem F, Waheed W, Gobbi M, et al. Preliminary evaluation of culturally sensitive CBT for Depression in Pakistan: Findings from developing culturally-sensitive CBT project (DCCP). Behav Cognit Psychother 2011;39(02):165–73.

60. Naeem F, Kingdon D, Saeed AA, et al. Urdu translation of the ICD-10 chapter V (F), Research Diagnostic Criteria (RDC): Process and principles of translation. Transcult Psychiatr 2011;48(4):484–95.

61. Rathod S, Phiri P, Harris S, et al. Cognitive behaviour therapy for psychosis can be adapted for minority ethnic groups: A randomised controlled trial. Schizophr Res 2013;143(2–3):319–26.

62. Naeem F, Saeed S, Irfan M, et al. Brief culturally adapted CBT for psychosis (CaCBTp): A randomized controlled trial from a low income country. Schizophr Res 2015;164(1):143–8.

63. Habib N, Dawood S, Kingdon D, et al. Preliminary evaluation of culturally adapted CBT for psychosis (CA-CBTp): findings from developing culturally-sensitive CBT Project (DCCP). Behav Cognit Psychother 2014. FirstView:1–9.

64. Husain MO, Chaudhry IB, Mehmood N, et al. Pilot randomised controlled trial of culturally adapted cognitive behavior therapy for psychosis (CaCBTp) in Pakistan. BMC Health Serv Res 2017;17(1):808.

65. Bhugra, Bhui Kamaldeep, Rosemarie MD. Cultural identity and its measurement: a questionnaire for Asians. Int Rev Psychiatr 1999;11(2–3):244–9.

66. Tam PWC, Wong DFK, Chow KKW, et al. Qualitative analysis of dysfunctional attitudes in Chinese persons suffering from depression. Hong Kong J Psychiatr 2007;17(4):109.

67. Lloyd KR, Jacob KS, Patel V, et al. The development of the short explanatory model interview (semi) and its use among primary-care attenders with common mental disorders. Psychol Med 1998;28(05):1231–7.

68. Testa S, Doucerain MM, Miglietta A, et al. The Vancouver Index of Acculturation (VIA): New evidence on dimensionality and measurement invariance across two cultural settings. Int J Intercult Relat 2019;71:60–71.

69. Weissman AN, Beck AT. Development and validation of the dysfunctional attitude scale: a preliminary investigation. 1978. Conference abstract; Annual Meeting of the American Educational Research Association, Toronto, Canada.

70. Rathod S, Kingdon D, Smith P, et al. Insight into Schizophrenia: the effects of cognitive behavioural therapy on the components of insight and association with sociodemographics—data on a previously published randomised controlled trial. Schizophr Res 2005;74(2–3):211–9.
71. Slingerland E. Body and mind in early china: an integrated humanities–science approach. J Am Acad Relig 2013;81(1):6–55.

A Review of Transdiagnostic Mechanisms in Cognitive Behavior Therapy

Matthew W. Southward, PhD*, Madeline L. Kushner, BA,
Douglas R. Terrill, MS, Shannon Sauer-Zavala, PhD

KEYWORDS

- Transdiagnostic • Mechanism • Cognitive behavior therapy • Skills • Alliance

KEY POINTS

- Transdiagnostic cognitive behavior therapies (CBTs) include CBT-specific skills, transtheoretical mechanisms, and psychopathological mechanisms.
- CBT-specific skills, such as cognitive restructuring or opposite-to-emotion action, may directly promote symptom reduction.
- Transtheoretical mechanisms, such as the alliance or treatment expectancies, may facilitate the efficacy of CBT-specific skills.
- Change in psychopathological mechanisms (eg, aversive reactivity, positive affectivity) may indicate subsequent symptom change.

A REVIEW OF TRANSDIAGNOSTIC MECHANISMS IN COGNITIVE BEHAVIOR THERAPY

Cognitive behavior therapy (CBT) is a psychological treatment in which patients are taught skills to regulate their emotions and more effectively manage their symptoms.[1] Relative to other forms of psychotherapy, CBT is brief, structured, and present-focused.[1] The cognitive behavioral approach is transdiagnostic,[2] having demonstrated efficacy in reducing symptoms for a wide range of psychiatric disorders.[3–5] It is important to note, however, that a substantial portion of patients (38%–65%) do not achieve full remission by the end of treatment.[3–5] To improve outcomes in CBT, it is important to identify active mechanisms of change during treatment[6] to ensure that CBTs engage these processes.

At least 3 classes of mechanisms outlined by Sauer-Zavala and colleagues[2] are relevant for psychological treatment (cf, Ref.[7] for other putative mechanisms). These

Department of Psychology, University of Kentucky, Lexington, KY, USA
* Corresponding author. Department of Psychology, University of Kentucky, 343 Waller Avenue, Suite 205, Lexington, KY 40504.
E-mail address: southward@uky.edu

Psychiatr Clin N Am 47 (2024) 343–354
https://doi.org/10.1016/j.psc.2024.02.003
0193-953X/24/© 2024 Elsevier Inc. All rights reserved.

classes can be characterized as treatment-specific therapeutic mechanisms thought to exert a direct impact on symptom change in specific CBTs, transtheoretical mechanisms thought to exert a broad impact on symptom change regardless of the treatment, and psychological mechanisms, thought to reflect changes in core psychological functioning signaling likely subsequent symptom changes. First, therapeutic mechanisms refer to the acquisition of competencies specific to a particular therapeutic approach; in skill-focused treatments such as CBT, the degree to which patients engage with the emotion regulation strategies taught may be an important driver of change.[8] Next, transtheoretical mechanisms (eg, working alliance, treatment expectancies) may facilitate improvement during all forms of psychotherapy, including CBT. Finally, psychopathological mechanisms refer to maladaptive, disorder-related processes that maintain symptoms (eg, experiential avoidance, negative affectivity); reductions in these processes may be necessary to observe symptom improvement. In this article, we review the evidence supporting these 3 classes of putative CBT mechanisms. We then discuss how these mechanisms may impact one another and provide recommendations for future psychotherapy treatment researchers to test these hypotheses.

Cognitive Behavior Therapy-specific Therapeutic Mechanisms

CBTs are designed to teach patients certain cognitive, behavioral, or mindfulness skills to more effectively manage their symptoms and promote more adaptive functioning. Cognitive skills involve identifying overly negative thoughts about oneself, other people, or the world and seeking out evidence to develop more balanced or realistic thoughts. Behavioral skills involve activities designed to provide new learning by challenging maladaptive urges to avoid emotions, people, or experiences that are less dangerous than one fears. Mindfulness and acceptance skills involve structured and experiential practices to cultivate nonjudgmental present-moment awareness of oneself and one's experiences. Other skills often taught in CBT but which do not fall cleanly into these categories include problem-solving, distraction, and social support. However, the cognitive, behavioral, and mindfulness skills used to manage daily stressors may be more impactful for a broader range of outcomes than these more specialized skills.[9]

In large-scale meta-analyses, some skills have demonstrated greater efficacy for certain outcomes than others. For instance, interoceptive exposure was associated with the largest improvements in panic disorder,[10] and behavioral activation was associated with the largest improvements in depression in Internet-delivered CBT[11] but not in-person CBT.[12] However, the fact that relatively few skills emerged as unique predictors of improvement for specific problems suggests that CBT skills may exert similarly sized effects on average across outcomes. Given that patients tend to use a wide range of skills in their daily lives,[13] the specific skills used may be less important to symptom changes than the order in which these skills are learned and specific aspects of how those skills are used.

Many CBTs are designed to teach patients skills in a prespecified order. However, patients typically present with a range of symptoms that may respond better to personalized sequences of skills. Researchers have begun to compare sequences of skills designed to capitalize on patients' pretreatment strengths to sequences designed to compensate for patients' pretreatment deficits. In general, sequences that capitalize on patients' strengths have demonstrated greater efficacy across a range of outcomes than those designed to compensate for patients' deficits ($g = .17$).[14] Recently, more comprehensive approaches to treatment personalization, such as process-based therapy (PBT), that advocate for idiographic tailoring in case conceptualization and progress tracking in addition to treatment selection and ordering[15] have begun to gain traction, though more research is necessary to determine the efficacy of doing so.

Southward and colleagues[16] developed a translational framework to delineate several potential aspects of skill use, including self-efficacy in using skills, the number of skills in patients' repertoires, how frequently patients use skills, and how well they use skills. Improvements in therapy skill self-efficacy have been associated with more frequent skill use,[17] predicted session-to-session reductions in panic symptoms,[18] and mediated the effect of CBT compared to waitlist on reductions in social anxiety.[19] Patients' skill repertoires may increase relatively linearly over treatment and those with larger repertoires tend to report fewer symptoms of anxiety and depression.[13] However, larger repertoires on a given day were associated with higher anxiety and lower depression among patients in a dialectical behavior therapy (DBT) skills group,[13] but predicted unique reductions in loneliness in the Unified Protocol (UP)[20] providing mixed evidence of the efficacy of skill repertoires as an active mechanism of treatment. By contrast, using therapy skills more frequently has predicted improvements in anxiety,[21,22] depression,[20–25] emotion dysregulation,[26] and distress tolerance[26] and mediated the effect of treatment on suicide attempts, nonsuicidal self-injury behaviors, anger expression, and depression.[27] Finally, higher quality skill use predicted decreases in depression across in-person[28] and Internet-delivered[29] cognitive therapy for depression. Self-reported skill quality also demonstrated the highest loading on a composite measure of skillfulness, and within-person changes in this composite measure predicted session-to-session reductions in anxiety and depression in the UP.[21]

Together, these results suggest that, beyond which skills patients use, beliefs in their abilities to use their skills, as well as the frequency and quality with which they use them may lead to the strongest and most consistent impact on a range of internalizing symptoms, whereas larger repertoires of skills may be less impactful on these outcomes. By also ordering the skills taught in treatment according to patients' pretreatment strengths, researchers may be able to further optimize the delivery of CBT for a range of conditions.

TRANSTHEORETICAL MECHANISMS
Working Alliance

One of the most well-studied transtheoretical mechanisms is the working alliance, defined as the collaborative relationship between patients and therapists.[30] Three distinct but related components are theorized to contribute to this relationship: agreement on the goals of the treatment; agreement on the specific tasks used to achieve these goals; and an emotional bond consisting of mutual respect and liking.[31] Patients who report a stronger alliance with their therapists tend to also report better treatment outcomes across a range of psychotherapies than patients who report a weaker alliance.[30]

Researchers have also observed within-person effects, which characterize how the strength of a patient's working alliance deviates from their personal average at any given session. Meta-analytically, within-person improvements in working alliance predicted subsequent session-to-session improvements in internalizing symptoms (eg, anxiety, depression, post-traumatic stress, and eating disorder symptoms; $\beta = -.07$).[32] These results held even when adjusting for concurrent treatment processes (eg, therapist compliance, homework compliance) and patient characteristics (eg, demographics, symptom severity), highlighting the robustness of the alliance-outcome association.[32]

In CBT, a positive alliance is often viewed as the context within which other techniques and skills can be most effectively used.[33] For example, within-person increases in the frequency of skill use mediated the effects of within-person increases in alliance on session-to-session reductions in depression among adolescents with depression receiving CBT.[34] Though limited, these results provide burgeoning empirical support for a facilitative effect of working alliance and skillfulness in producing session-to-session symptom change.

Treatment Expectancies

Similar to the alliance, expectations for treatment can influence patients' engagement in and success with therapy. Expectations demonstrated a small-to-medium-sized meta-analytic association with posttreatment outcomes ($r = 0.18$).[35] Treatment credibility, or patients' perception of how suitable a treatment seems, has similarly been associated with treatment outcomes, with small-to-moderate effect sizes (ηs: -0.18–-0.25).[36] Although there is some debate over whether expectations and credibility represent the same process, patients often form expectations prior to gaining any significant information regarding the treatment.[37] Thus, although conceptually similar, expectations and credibility are considered distinct constructs that both contribute to successful treatment.[38]

Self-efficacy

Patient factors have also been considered as possible mechanisms by which change in therapy occurs. Self-efficacy is conceptualized as patients' beliefs that they can successfully execute behaviors necessary to produce change.[39] If patients believe that they can effectively use CBT skills in their daily lives, they are more likely to try to do so. Self-efficacy beliefs have been proposed to be a transdiagnostic mechanism of change and play a role in the development of anxiety.[40] Indeed, in CBT for social anxiety disorder, improvements in self-efficacy mediated the effect of CBT on social anxiety symptoms and were associated with lower social anxiety symptoms at 1 year followup.[19] In CBT for panic disorder, increases in self-efficacy were found to temporally precede changes in panic symptoms, indicating that changes in self-efficacy influence subsequent symptom changes.[18] Taken together, these results suggest that increased self-efficacy may serve as a mechanism by which symptom change occurs in CBT.

Overall, each of these transtheoretical mechanisms may contribute to change, regardless of the psychotherapy administered. Of course, all of these mechanisms likely contribute to successful therapy, and the extent to which each mechanism facilitates change varies from patient to patient.[41] Still, continued investigation into general mechanisms of change is necessary, as more clarity in this area will help researchers and clinicians improve the efficacy of psychotherapy.

PSYCHOPATHOLOGICAL MECHANISMS

CBT may be most efficacious for internalizing disorders such as anxiety, depressive, eating, and related disorders.[7] Thus, in the following section, we review psychopathological processes thought to maintain internalizing disorders, along with the evidence that CBTs engage these targets.

Aversive Reactivity

Aversive reactivity denotes the perception of negative emotions as uncontrollable, intolerable, dangerous, or unacceptable.[42] This broad construct has been referred to as anxiety sensitivity, experiential avoidance, intolerance of uncertainty, negative urgency, and distress intolerance,[43] though these processes may all represent a unified factor.[44] Barlow and colleagues[45,46] describe aversive reactivity as a functional mechanism implicated in the development and maintenance of internalizing disorders. When negative emotional experiences, common in people with internalizing psychopathology, are met with aversive reactions, patients are more likely to engage in avoidant coping behaviors (ie, attempts to dampen, control, or escape negative emotions). Though emotional avoidance may provide momentary relief from negative affect, these behaviors exacerbate negative affect in the long term; this creates a positive feedback loop leading to the development and/or worsening of emotional disorder symptoms.[47]

There is burgeoning evidence that aversive reactivity is a putative mechanism of change in treatments for internalizing disorders. Reductions in aversive reactivity accounted for improvements in internalizing symptoms and were associated with increases in well-being in the UP.[44,48,49] Decreases in aversive reactivity also preceded and predicted improvements in emotional disorder symptoms among patients receiving a range of CBT protocols, and a number of specific CBT strategies (eg, mindfulness training, cognitive restructuring, exposures) are associated with improvements in aversive reactivity.[50,51]

Together, the literature on aversive reactivity suggests that how one relates to negative emotions is an important predictor of psychological health, even beyond the experience of negative emotions alone.[49] Moreover, preliminary evidence suggests that CBT protocols, as well as specific strategies drawn from CBT, may address aversive reactivity. However, most researchers have only investigated specific forms of aversive reactivity. We encourage future researchers to develop and validate a comprehensive measure of this construct that can be used across diagnoses and treatment protocols to more directly test its mechanistic effects during CBT.

Positive Affectivity

Existing treatments for emotional disorders have primarily focused on reducing or improving how people cope with negative affect, rather than enhancing positive affect. High positive affect is associated with greater well-being, physical health, and resilience,[52] whereas low positive affect has been implicated in the onset and maintenance of a range of emotional disorders.[53]

Improvements in positive affect have mediated improvements in depression and predicted changes in social anxiety over the course of mindfulness-based cognitive therapy (MBCT)[54] suggesting that changes in positive affect may be a mechanism of MBCT.[55] Several positive psychology interventions that are similar to CBT approaches (eg, savoring, cultivating and expressing gratitude, engaging in acts of kindness, and pursuit of hope and meaning in life) have improved well-being and reduced depressive symptoms,[56] although it remains unclear whether these interventions improve positive affect.[57] Recently, 2 novel CBTs developed to target anhedonia by enhancing positive affect, behavioral activation for the treatment of anhedonia[58] and positive affect treatment,[59] have improved positive affect and reduced anxiety, depression, and suicidal ideation.[58,60,61]

By contrast, bipolar disorder is marked by abnormally persistent positive or elevated moods during periods of mania.[62] Some have argued that excess positive affect in bipolar disorder is best addressed using medication,[63] perhaps contributing to the limited number of behavioral interventions focused on the downregulation of positive affectivity. GOALS, a therapeutic intervention centered on preventing manic episodes by reducing the setting and pursuit of overly ambitious goals is one exception, though additional research is necessary to confirm its efficacy.[64] In addition, interpersonal and social rhythm therapy, which aims to stabilize positive affect by tracking one's emotions and activities which alter mood (eg, sleep, interpersonal factors), has demonstrated efficacy in extending periods between manic episodes.[65]

In sum, there is some evidence of positive affectivity as a transdiagnostic mechanism of CBT, and results of early trials testing novel comprehensive positive affect interventions have demonstrated meaningful reductions in emotional disorder symptoms. We encourage future researchers to test whether changes in positive affectivity predict subsequent symptom changes in these therapies to enhance these initial findings. Incorporating positive affect as a treatment target into existing CBT protocols may augment their efficacy by simultaneously downregulating negative affect and upregulating positive affect.

Attachment Style

In attachment theory, the responsiveness of caregivers, friends, and colleagues is thought to shape our interpersonal behaviors, cognitions, and emotions.[66,67] Insecure attachment styles (ie, ambivalent, avoidant, disorganized) are thought to result from close others who are inconsistent or unavailable in responding to a person's needs.[68] People with insecure attachment styles may feel vulnerable in relationships, which can manifest as excessive fear of rejection and panic when confronted with the possibility of abandonment or, conversely, as an antagonistic disposition and exaggerated distrust toward others.[69] Insecure attachment styles are over-represented among those with emotional disorders, highlighting its transdiagnostic relevancy.[69–71]

Evidence-based treatments targeting attachment insecurity include interpersonal psychotherapy[72] and attachment-based family therapy.[73] Reductions in attachment anxiety and avoidance during these treatments have been associated with reductions in depression, though it remains unclear whether there is a causal relation between these two constructs. Borderline personality disorder (BPD) Compass, a personality-based CBT for BPD, is designed to engage attachment insecurity as a functional mechanism linking temperamental antagonism to externalizing symptoms.[74,75] BPD Compass includes evidence-based methods to improve attachment insecurity, such as coaching patients to consider others' perspective and modifying negative beliefs about others' trustworthiness, with the goal of reducing antagonism.

Other cognitive behavioral interventions do not explicitly target insecure attachment in name, though some may indirectly address it. DBT,[76] for instance, includes assertiveness training which teaches skills for expressing one's needs in a confident and polite manner. Schema-focused therapy[77] challenges maladaptive patterns of thinking and feeling (ie, schemas) about relationships using cognitive therapy techniques. Both treatments have improved interpersonal functioning among patients with BPD.[78,79] Although CBT researchers have not often studied attachment insecurity as a mechanism of change, evidence of its transdiagnostic relevance, malleability in treatment, and associations with symptom reduction warrant further inquiry.

SUMMARY AND FUTURE DIRECTIONS

Engaging mechanisms responsible for change during CBT is important for increasing the potency and efficiency of our interventions. By ensuring that all strategies included in CBTs improve putative therapeutic, transtheoretical, and/or psychopathological mechanisms, treatment developers may be able to distill their interventions down to only active ingredients. In this article, we reviewed the roles that (1) CBT-specific skill competencies (therapeutic mechanisms), (2) general treatment factors (transtheoretical mechanisms), and (3) disorder-related processes that maintain symptoms (psychopathological mechanisms) play in enacting symptom improvement during CBT.

In general, there is good support for the association between most of the proposed putative mechanisms for CBT and psychological symptoms. Specifically, deficits in CBT skills (eg, low levels of mindfulness), psychopathological processes (eg, high levels of aversive reactivity), and common factors (eg, a limited bond with one's therapists) are transdiagnostically associated with a range of mental health conditions. There is also strong support that CBT-specific skill competencies, such as cognitive flexibility, behavior change, and mindfulness, improve during cognitive behavioral interventions. Although relatively fewer researchers have examined changes in transtheoretical processes, there is emerging evidence that these processes, particularly the alliance, also fluctuate and improve during CBT. The degree of support for putative psychopathological mechanisms improving throughout treatment is variable, with some processes (eg, aversive reactivity, positive affectivity) demonstrating change across multiple studies, and others (eg, attachment security) having been tested in relatively fewer trials.

Demonstrating that a construct is associated with psychopathology and improves during treatment is a preliminary step in identifying putative mechanisms, but more evidence is needed to determine whether improvement in a particular construct is driving any observed symptom change.[6] Only recently have researchers been collecting data on putative mechanisms and outcomes with enough frequency to draw conclusions about temporal precedence (ie, does change in the hypothesized mechanism precede and predict change in the outcome?). Future treatment outcome researchers should conduct intensive, longitudinal data collections to parse how changes in variables of interest interact across time. However, even when temporal precedence for a putative mechanism can be inferred, the amount of variance in the outcome explained by the mediating construct is often small in magnitude. It is thus likely that multiple processes contribute to symptom improvement during CBT. When assessing these multiple processes, we encourage future researchers to explore main effects, mediating effects, and moderating effects of these processes on one another to predict symptom outcomes, using theoretical considerations as a guide (eg, CBT skill use mediating the effect of the alliance on depression symptom change outcomes).[34] We encourage future mechanistic researchers to take advantage of more sophisticated analytical tools (eg, longitudinal network modeling; multilevel structural equation modeling) that can accommodate relations among multiple candidate processes. Additionally, it may be possible to design treatment studies that directly manipulate mechanistic processes to draw more robust causal conclusions about their effects on treatment outcomes.[8]

The PBT framework, mentioned earlier, may be particularly amenable to the manipulation of mechanistic processes as it specifies particular process of change that may be active and targeted in treatment.[80] By testing how the mechanisms that maintain symptoms vary across patients, including those who receive the same diagnosis or therapy, the PBT framework can allow for fruitful research into both general and unique mechanisms of change in treatment.[81] By studying these mechanisms at a dynamic level as they unfold and impact one another over time, researchers can leverage advanced analytical methods to identify how the effects of these putative mechanisms may change over the course of treatment of specific patients.[82]

Taken together, there is a growing foundation of research on processes of change in CBT. It is likely that increases in therapeutic skills, decreases in maladaptive psychopathological processes, and transtheoretical factors all contribute to symptom improvement during a course of CBT. However, to be more confident that these factors *drive* change in CBT, and to better represent a reality in which multiple constructs likely interact to produce symptom improvement, future researchers must take advantage of innovative trial designs and sophisticated analytical techniques. Continuing to invest resources in understanding mechanisms of change in psychotherapy is paramount for increasing the potency and parsimony of our protocols with the aim of improving outcomes.

CLINICS CARE POINTS

- Helping patients use cognitive, behavioral, and mindfulness skills more frequently and more skillfully may directly promote improvements in anxiety and depression.
- Generating buy-in for the use of these skills by clearly demonstrating how they can be used to address patients' primary concerns can facilitate patients' skill frequency and quality.
- Helping patients understand that emotions are informative and not dangerous relatively early in treatment may help reduce aversive reactions to those emotions and facilitate subsequent reductions in anxiety and depression.

DISCLOSURE

S. Sauer-Zavala receives royalties from the Oxford University Press in her role as an author of the Unified Protocol. M.W. Southward's efforts on this paper were partially supported by the National Institute of Mental Health, United States under award number K23MH126211. The content is solely the responsibility of the author and does not necessarily represent the official views of the National Institute of Health.

REFERENCES

1. Beck JS. Cognitive behavior therapy: basics and beyond. 2nd edition. New York, NY: Guilford; 2011.
2. Sauer-Zavala S, Gutner CA, Farchione TJ, et al. Current definitions of "transdiagnostic" in treatment development: A search for consensus. Behav Ther 2017; 48(1):128–38.
3. Cuijpers P, Karyotaki E, Weitz E, et al. The effects of psychotherapies for major depression in adults on remission, recovery and improvement: A meta-analysis. J Affect Disord 2014;159:118–26.
4. Springer KS, Levy HC, Tolin DF. Remission in CBT for adult anxiety disorders: A meta-analysis. Clin Psychol Rev 2018;61:1–8.
5. Zanarini MC, Frankenburg FR, Reich DB, et al. Attainment and stability of sustained symptomatic remission and recovery among patients with borderline personality disorder and axis II comparison subjects: A 16-year prospective follow-up study. Am J Psychiatry 2012;169(5):476–83.
6. Kazdin AE. Mediators and mechanisms of change in psychotherapy research. Annu Rev Clin Psychol 2007;3:1–27.
7. Kazantzis N, Luong HK, Usatoff AS, et al. The processes of cognitive behavioral therapy: A review of meta-analyses. Cogn Ther Res 2018;42:349–57.
8. Southward MW, Sauer-Zavala S. Experimental manipulations to test theory-driven mechanisms of cognitive behavior therapy. Front Psychiatry 2020;11:603009.
9. Cheavens JS, Southward MW, Howard KP, et al. Broad strokes or fine points: Are dialectical behavior therapy modules associated with general or domain-specific changes? Personal Disord 2023;14(2):137–47.
10. Pompoli A, Furukawa TA, Efthimiou O, et al. Dismantling cognitive-behaviour therapy for panic disorder: a systematic review and component network meta-analysis. Psychol Med 2018;48(12):1945–53.

11. Furukawa TA, Suganuma A, Ostinelli EG, et al. Dismantling, optimising, and personalising internet cognitive behavioural therapy for depression: a systematic review and component network meta-analysis using individual participant data. Lancet Psychiatr 2021;8(6):500–11.

12. López-López JA, Davies SR, Caldwell DM, et al. The process and delivery of CBT for depression in adults: a systematic review and network meta-analysis. Psychol Med 2019;49(12):1937–47.

13. Southward MW, Eberle JW, Neacsiu AD. Multilevel associations of daily skill use and effectiveness with anxiety, depression, and stress in a transdiagnostic sample undergoing dialectical behavior therapy skills training. Cognit Behav Ther 2022;51(2):114–29.

14. Flückiger C, Munder T, Del Re AC, et al. Strength-based methods - a narrative review and comparative multilevel meta-analysis of positive interventions in clinical settings. Psychother Res 2023;33(7):856–72.

15. Ong CW, Hayes SC, Hofmann SG. A process-based approach to cognitive behavioral therapy: A theory-based case illustration. Front Psychol 2022;13:1002849.

16. Southward MW, Sauer-Zavala S, Cheavens JS. Specifying the mechanisms and targets of emotion regulation: A translational framework from affective science to psychological treatment. Clin Psychol 2021;28(2):168–82.

17. Barnicot K, Gonzalez R, McCabe R, et al. Skills use and common treatment processes in dialectical behaviour therapy for borderline personality disorder. J Behav Ther Exp Psychiatry 2016;52:147–56.

18. Gallagher MW, Payne LA, White KS, et al. Mechanisms of change in cognitive behavioral therapy for panic disorder: the unique effects of self-efficacy and anxiety sensitivity. Behav Res Ther 2013;51(11):767–77.

19. Goldin PR, Ziv M, Jazaieri H, et al. Cognitive reappraisal self-efficacy mediates the effects of individual cognitive-behavioral therapy for social anxiety disorder. J Consult Clin Psychol 2012;80(6):1034–40.

20. Southward MW, Terrill DR, Sauer-Zavala S. The effects of the Unified Protocol and Unified Protocol skills on loneliness in the COVID-19 pandemic. Depress Anxiety 2022;39(12):913–21.

21. Southward MW, Sauer-Zavala S. Dimensions of skill use in the unified protocol: Exploring unique effects on anxiety and depression. J Consult Clin Psychol 2022;90(3):246–57.

22. Webb CA, Beard C, Kertz SJ, et al. Differential role of CBT skills, DBT skills and psychological flexibility in predicting depressive versus anxiety symptom improvement. Behav Res Ther 2016;81:12–20.

23. Radkovsky A, McArdle JJ, Bockting CL, et al. Successful emotion regulation skills application predicts subsequent reduction of symptom severity during treatment of major depressive disorder. J Consult Clin Psychol 2014;82(2):248–62.

24. Webb CA, Stanton CH, Bondy E, et al. Cognitive versus behavioral skills in CBT for depressed adolescents: Disaggregating within-patient versus between-patient effects on symptom change. J Consult Clin Psychol 2019;87(5):484–90.

25. Wirtz CM, Radkovsky A, Ebert DD, et al. Successful application of adaptive emotion regulation skills predicts the subsequent reduction of depressive symptom severity but neither the reduction of anxiety nor the reduction of general distress during the treatment of major depressive disorder. PLoS One 2014;9(10):e108288.

26. Southward MW, Howard KP, Cheavens JS. Less is more: Decreasing the frequency of maladaptive coping predicts improvements in DBT more consistently

than increasing the frequency of adaptive coping. Behav Res Ther 2023;163: 104288.

27. Neacsiu AD, Rizvi SL, Linehan MM. Dialectical behavior therapy skills use as a mediator and outcome of treatment for borderline personality disorder. Behav Res Ther 2010;48(9):832–9.

28. Strunk DR, Hollars SN, Adler AD, et al. Assessing Patients' Cognitive Therapy Skills: Initial Evaluation of the Competencies of Cognitive Therapy Scale. Cognit Ther Res 2014;38(5):559–69.

29. Forand NR, Barnett JG, Strunk DR, et al. Efficacy of Guided iCBT for Depression and Mediation of Change by Cognitive Skill Acquisition. Behav Ther 2018;49(2): 295–307.

30. Flückiger C, Del Re AC, Wampold BE, et al. The alliance in adult psychotherapy: A meta-analytic synthesis. Psychotherapy 2018;55(4):316–40.

31. Bordin ES. The generalizability of the psychoanalytic concept of the working alliance. Psychol Psychother 1979;16(3):252–60.

32. Flückiger C, Rubel J, Del Re AC, et al. The reciprocal relationship between alliance and early treatment symptoms: A two-stage individual participant data meta-analysis. J Consult Clin Psychol 2020;88(9):829–43.

33. Goldfried MR, Davila J. The role of relationship and technique in therapeutic change. Psychotherapy 2005;42(4):421–30.

34. Lindqvist K, Mechler J, Falkenström F, et al. Therapeutic alliance is calming and curing-The interplay between alliance and emotion regulation as predictors of outcome in Internet-based treatments for adolescent depression. J Consult Clin Psychol 2023;91(7):426–37.

35. Constantino MJ, Vîslă A, Coyne AE, et al. A meta-analysis of the association between patients' early treatment outcome expectation and their posttreatment outcomes. Psychotherapy (Chic) 2018;55(4):473–85.

36. Mooney TK, Gibbons MB, Gallop R, et al. Psychotherapy credibility ratings: patient predictors of credibility and the relation of credibility to therapy outcome. Psychother Res 2014;24(5):565–77.

37. Schulte D. Patients' outcome expectancies and their impression of suitability as predictors of treatment outcome. Psychother Res 2008;18(4):481–94.

38. Panitz C, Endres D, Buchholz M, et al. A Revised Framework for the Investigation of Expectation Update Versus Maintenance in the Context of Expectation Violations: The VioIEx 2.0 Model. Front Psychol 2021;12:726432.

39. Bandura A. Self-efficacy: toward a unifying theory of behavioral change. Psychol Rev 1977;84(2):191–215.

40. Bandura A. Self-efficacy conception of anxiety. In: Schwarzer R, Wicklund RA, editors. Anxiety and self-focused attention. Harwood: London, UK: Academic Publishers; 1991. p. 89–110.

41. Antichi L, Giannini M. An introduction to change in psychotherapy: Moderators, course of change, and change mechanisms. J Contemp Psychother 2023. https://doi.org/10.1007/s10879-023-09590-x.

42. Sauer-Zavala S, Southward MW, Semcho SA. Integrating and differentiating personality and psychopathology in cognitive behavioral therapy. J Pers 2022;90(1): 89–102.

43. Semcho SA, Southward MW, Stumpp NE, et al. Aversive reactivity: A transdiagnostic functional bridge between neuroticism and avoidant behavioral coping. J Emotion Psychopathol 2023;1(1):23–40.

44. Semcho SA, Southward MW, Stumpp NE, et al. Within-person changes in aversive reactivity predict session-to-session reductions in anxiety and depression

in the unified protocol [published online ahead of print, 2023 Sep 13]. Psychother Res 2023;1–14. https://doi.org/10.1080/10503307.2023.2254467.

45. Barlow DH, Sauer-Zavala S, Carl JR, et al. The nature, diagnosis, and treatment of neuroticism: Back to the future. Clin Psychol Sci 2014;2(3):344–65.

46. Bullis JR, Boettcher H, Sauer-Zavala S, et al. What is an emotional disorder? A transdiagnostic mechanistic definition with implications for assessment, treatment, and prevention. Clin Psychol 2019;26(2):e12278.

47. Abramowitz JS, Tolin DF, Street GP. Paradoxical effects of thought suppression: a meta-analysis of controlled studies. Clin Psychol Rev 2001;21(5):683–703.

48. Elhusseini SA, Cravens LE, Southward MW, et al. Associations between improvements in aversive reactions to negative emotions and increased quality of life in the Unified Protocol. J Behav Cogn Ther 2022;32(1):25–32.

49. Sauer-Zavala S, Boswell JF, Gallagher MW, et al. The role of negative affectivity and negative reactivity to emotions in predicting outcomes in the Unified Protocol for the transdiagnostic treatment of emotional disorders. Behav Res Ther 2012; 50(9):551–7.

50. Alimehdi M, Ehteshamzadeh P, Naderi F, et al. The effectiveness of mindfulness-based stress reduction on intolerance of uncertainty and anxiety sensitivity among individuals with generalized anxiety disorder. Asian Soc Sci 2016;12(4): Article 4.

51. Eustis EH, Cardona N, Nauphal M, et al. Experiential avoidance as a mechanism of change across cognitive-behavioral therapy in a sample of participants with heterogeneous anxiety disorders. Cogn Ther Res 2020;44(2):275–86.

52. Cohen S, Pressman SD. Positive affect and health. Curr Dir Psychol 2006;15(3): 122–5.

53. Brown TA. Temporal course and structural relationships among dimensions of temperament and DSM-IV anxiety and mood disorder constructs. J Abnorm Psychol 2007;116(2):313–28.

54. Segal ZV, Williams JMG, Teasdale JD. Mindfulness-based cognitive therapy for depression. 1st edition. New York, NY: Guilford; 2001.

55. Batink T, Peeters F, Geschwind N, et al. How does MBCT for depression work? studying cognitive and affective mediation pathways. PLoS One 2013;8(8): e72778.

56. Sin NL, Lyubomirsky S. Enhancing well-being and alleviating depressive symptoms with positive psychology interventions: a practice-friendly meta-analysis. J Clin Psychol 2009;65(5):467–87.

57. Moskowitz JT, Cheung EO, Freedman M, et al. Measuring positive emotion outcomes in positive psychology interventions: A literature review. Emotion Rev 2021;13(1):60–73.

58. Cernasov P, Walsh EC, Kinard JL, et al. Multilevel growth curve analyses of behavioral activation for anhedonia (BATA) and mindfulness-based cognitive therapy effects on anhedonia and resting-state functional connectivity: Interim results of a randomized trial. J Affect Disord 2021;292:161–71.

59. Craske MG, Meuret AE, Ritz T, et al. Treatment for Anhedonia: A Neuroscience Driven Approach. Depress Anxiety 2016;33(10):927–38.

60. Craske MG, Meuret AE, Ritz T, et al. Positive affect treatment for depression and anxiety: A randomized clinical trial for a core feature of anhedonia. J Consult Clin Psychol 2019;87(5):457–71.

61. Phillips R, Walsh E, Cernasov P, et al. Concurrent reduction in anhedonia severity and self-reported stress following psychotherapy treatment for transdiagnostic anhedonia. Biol Psychiatry 2021;89(9):S327–8.

62. American Psychiatric Association. Diagnostic and statistical manual of mental disorders: DSM-5. Washington, DC: American Psychiatric Association; 2013.

63. Nivoli AM, Murru A, Goikolea JM, et al. New treatment guidelines for acute bipolar mania: a critical review. J Affect Disord 2012;140(2):125–41.

64. Johnson SL, Fulford D. Preventing mania: a preliminary examination of the GOALS Program. Behav Ther 2009;40(2):103–13.

65. Frank E, Kupfer DJ, Thase ME, et al. Two-year outcomes for interpersonal and social rhythm therapy in individuals with bipolar I disorder. Arch Gen Psychiatry 2005;62(9):996–1004.

66. Bowlby J. Attachment and loss: attachment. New York, NY: Basic Books; 1969.

67. Chopik WJ, Edelstein RS, Grimm KJ. Longitudinal changes in attachment orientation over a 59-year period. J Pers Soc Psychol 2019;116(4):598–611.

68. Ainsworth MDS, Blehar MC, Waters E, et al. Patterns of attachment: a psychological study of the strange situation. New York, NY: Lawrence Erlbaum; 1978.

69. Herstell S, Betz LT, Penzel N, et al. Insecure attachment as a transdiagnostic risk factor for major psychiatric conditions: A meta-analysis in bipolar disorder, depression and schizophrenia spectrum disorder. J Psychiatr Res 2021;144: 190–201.

70. Lorenzini N, Fonagy P. Attachment and personality disorders: A short review. FOCUS 2013;11(2):155–66.

71. Woodhouse S, Ayers S, Field AP. The relationship between adult attachment style and post-traumatic stress symptoms: A meta-analysis. J Anxiety Disord 2015;35: 103–17.

72. Weissman MM, Markowitz JC, Klerman G. Comprehensive guide to interpersonal psychotherapy. New York, NY: Basic Books; 2008.

73. Diamond GS, Diamond GM, Levy SA. Attachment-based family therapy for depressed adolescents. Washington, DC: American Psychological Association; 2014.

74. Sauer-Zavala S, Southward MW, Fruhbauerova M, et al. BPD compass: A randomized controlled trial of a short-term, personality-based treatment for borderline personality disorder. Personal Disord 2023;14(5):534–44.

75. Sauer-Zavala S, Southward MW, Hood CO, et al. Conceptual development and case data for a modular, personality-based treatment for borderline personality disorder. Personal Disord 2023;14(4):369–80.

76. Linehan MM. Cognitive-behavioral treatment of borderline personality disorder. New York, NY: Guilford Press; 1993.

77. Young JE, Klosko JS, Weishaar ME. Schema therapy: a practitioner's guide. New York, NY: Guilford Press; 2003.

78. Bamelis LL, Evers SM, Spinhoven P, et al. Results of a multicenter randomized controlled trial of the clinical effectiveness of schema therapy for personality disorders. Am J Psychiatry 2014;171(3):305–22.

79. Swenson CR, Sanderson C, Dulit RA, et al. The application of dialectical behavior therapy for patients with borderline personality disorder on inpatient units. Psychiatr Q 2001;72(4):307–24.

80. Hofmann SG, Hayes SC. The future of intervention science: Process-based therapy. Clin Psychol Sci 2019;7(1):37–50.

81. Hayes SC, Hofmann SG, Stanton CE, et al. The role of the individual in the coming era of process-based therapy. Behav Res Ther 2019;117:40–53.

82. Hofmann SG, Curtiss JE, Hayes SC. Beyond linear mediation: Toward a dynamic network approach to study treatment processes. Clin Psychol Rev 2020;76: 101824.

Cognitive-Behavioral Therapy Enhancement Strategies

David F. Tolin, PhD[a,b],*, Kayla A. Lord, PhD[a], Kelly A. Knowles, PhD[a]

KEYWORDS

- Cognitive-behavioral therapy • Pharmacotherapy • D-cycloserine • Exercise
- Transcranial magnetic stimulation

KEY POINTS

- Traditional pharmacotherapy has only a small benefit when added to CBT for anxiety and depression.
- D-cycloserine may enhance or accelerate CBT results.
- Exercise appears to enhance CBT results.
- It is unclear whether noninvasive brain stimulation augments CBT results.
- Other compounds of interest await controlled research.

INTRODUCTION

The efficacy of cognitive-behavioral therapy (CBT) for anxiety and depressive disorders is well documented. Randomized controlled trials (RCTs) have demonstrated that CBT is superior to control conditions in the treatment of panic disorder, generalized anxiety disorder, social anxiety disorder (SAD), obsessive-compulsive disorder (OCD), and posttraumatic stress disorder (PTSD),[1] as well as major depressive disorder (MDD) and persistent depressive disorder.[2] However, it is also clear that there is substantial room for improvement in these treatments. Across studies of anxiety disorders, only half of the patients are classified as treatment responders.[3] Across studies of depressive disorders, response rates are even lower at 42%.[4] Thus, although CBT is efficacious, half or more of patients with anxiety or depressive disorders do not show a favorable response. In this article, we will describe efforts to augment CBT with biological interventions, the available evidence on whether these enhancements boost CBT's efficacy, and promising directions for future research.

a The Institute of Living/Hartford Hospital, 200 Retreat Avenue, Hartford, CT 06106, USA; b Yale University School of Medicine
* Corresponding author. Anxiety Disorders Center, The Institute of Living, 200 Retreat Avenue, Hartford, CT 06106.
E-mail address: david.tolin@hhchealth.org

Psychiatr Clin N Am 47 (2024) 355–365
https://doi.org/10.1016/j.psc.2024.02.005
0193-953X/24/© 2024 Elsevier Inc. All rights reserved.

psych.theclinics.com

TRADITIONAL PHARMACOTHERAPY

Traditional pharmacotherapy for anxiety and depressive disorders includes antide-pressants, such as selective serotonin reuptake inhibitors, and benzodiazepines and azapirones; these treatments have been shown to be reasonably efficacious monotherapies, with small to medium effects[5,6] that may be more readily detected in severe cases.[7] Meta-analysis demonstrates that combined treatment (CBT + pharmacotherapy) is significantly better than CBT alone although the effects are small for antidepressants, and there was no evidence of a facilitative effect of ben-zodiazepines.[8] Furthermore, some evidence suggests that the long-term effects of combined therapy may be worse than those of CBT alone.[9,10] Thus, although tradi-tional pharmacotherapy (particularly antidepressants) may augment CBT, this is far from an ideal solution, and additional strategies are clearly needed.

PRINCIPLES FOR A NEW PARADIGM OF COGNITIVE-BEHAVIORAL THERAPY ENHANCEMENT

An exciting line of research has developed over the past 2 decades that investigates the biological mechanisms of CBT and identifies compounds that target and poten-tiate those mechanisms. Rather than augmentation where two successful monothera-pies are combined, this augmentation strategy does not presuppose that the augmenting compound has anxiolytic or antidepressant properties by itself; instead, biologic agents are selected based on their capacity to enhance the mechanisms of CBT. To date, most of this work has been conducted in the anxiety-related disorders, largely because *fear extinction* mechanisms can be easily identified and studied in both animals and humans.[11]

To determine whether an augmenting intervention enhances CBT, researchers must compare combined treatment (CBT + enhancer) to CBT monotherapy (CBT + placebo) in a RCT. While there are several intriguing open trials of potential augmenting interventions, one cannot infer efficacy from these trials. As such, in this article, we will focus on RCTs comparing combined treatment to placebo-augmented CBT monotherapy.

D-CYCLOSERINE

Fear extinction is controlled, in part, by glutamatergic activity at the N-methyl D-ethyl aspartate (NMDA) receptor, which is particularly concentrated in basolateral amyg-dala.[12] The antibiotic D-cycloserine (DCS), which has no inherent anxiolytic properties, acts as a partial agonist of the NMDA receptor and has been demonstrated to poten-tiate the extinction of conditioned fear in rats.[13] This finding led to human trials of exposure-based CBT for anxiety-related disorders. RCTs of (CBT + DCS) versus (CBT + placebo) showed a beneficial effect of DCS in patients with specific phobia,[14,15] panic disorder,[16] OCD,[17,18] and SAD.[19] Further evidence suggests that DCS augmentation may be maximally effective when administered after a session of exposure therapy, suggesting action in the consolidation phase of fear extinction.[20] The success of postexposure administration of DCS also appears to be contingent on the success of the exposure session: When DCS is administered after a "successful" exposure in which the patient's fear subsided during the session, DCS's effects are substantially stronger than those when administered after an "unsuccessful" session in which fear did not subside[21,22] although a tailored approach was not superior to fixed dosing in a randomized trial.[23] Across RCTs of DCS, the facilitative effect of DCS appears to be small[24]; however, the body of work on DCS serves as proof of concept that a psychiatrically inert agent can be used to potentiate the biological mechanisms of CBT.

EXERCISE

As a monotherapy, exercise yields large effects on depressive symptoms[25] and moderate effects on anxiety.[26] Several biological mechanisms may explain how exercise improves psychological functioning, such as through the hypothalamic-pituitary-adrenal axis and circulation of glucocorticoids,[27] upregulation of the brain-derived neurotrophic factor (BDNF),[28] and reduced inflammation.[29] Psychological mechanisms may also account for the beneficial effects of exercise on mood and anxiety disorders, as exercise can serve as behavioral activation, reducing depressive symptoms,[30] and may teach individuals not to fear bodily sensations, reducing anxiety sensitivity.[31]

Several RCTs have examined CBT + exercise compared to CBT alone or with an educational control group. For example, a recent pilot study found large improvements in anhedonia among depressed individuals who exercised before CBT sessions compared to those who did not, as well as a moderate improvement in overall depressive symptoms at 3-month follow-up.[32] In another study, depressed outpatients who received group CBT with three weekly group exercise classes reported greater decreases in depressive symptoms, suicidal ideation, and disability compared to those who received CBT alone,[33] extending the benefits of exercise beyond mere symptom change. Among individuals with anxiety disorders, patients who received group CBT and exercise encouragement experienced greater declines in depression, anxiety, and stress scores than did those who received CBT + nutritional education;[34] those who made improvements in their level of activity, regardless of group allocation, had the highest mean changes in depression, anxiety, and stress. Finally, a promising pilot study found that individuals with PTSD who participated in 30 minutes of moderate-intensity exercise before prolonged exposure (PE) therapy sessions demonstrated greater improvement in their PTSD symptoms and greater BDNF compared to those who received PE alone,[28] supporting increased BDNF as a potential mechanism of the adjunctive effect of exercise.

NONINVASIVE BRAIN STIMULATION

Despite widespread interest in noninvasive brain stimulation (NIBS) as a psychotherapeutic enhancer,[35] empirical findings are mixed. NIBS involves applying a magnetic field, as in transcranial magnetic stimulation (TMS), or weak electrical current, as in transcranial direct current stimulation (tDCS), over the scalp, which enhances the metabolism of the targeted brain area, thereby modifying brain functions.[36] The impact of NIBS depends on the intensity and frequency of stimulation and the targeted area, typically the prefrontal cortex (PFC).

RCTs of CBT + active TMS versus CBT + sham TMS have demonstrated limited augmenting effects. In support of an augmenting effect, mindfulness-based stress reduction for poststroke depression + repetitive TMS (rTMS) over the left dorsolateral PFC (DLPFC) enhanced all clinical outcomes,[37] and deep TMS (dTMS) over the medial PFC and anterior cingulate cortex following exposure to feared stimuli reduced OCD symptoms more than did sham TMS.[38] In addition, while exposure + medial PFC dTMS for PTSD was related to decreased intrusion symptoms in a pilot trial,[39] in a multicenter RCT of imaginal exposure + medial PFC dTMS for PTSD, dTMS *attenuated* symptom reduction.[40] Another pilot trial found that PE + rTMS was feasible with a nonsignificant trend toward improvement in PTSD symptoms, but power was insufficient to detect between-group effects.[41] Furthermore, left PFC intermittent theta burst stimulation, a specific type of TMS, did not augment CBT for panic disorder[42,43] nor virtual reality exposure for arachnophobia.[44,45] Of note, in an RCT using a transdiagnostic framework (ie, all participants had at least one diagnosis according to the Diagnostic and Statistical Manual of Mental Disorders, 5th Edition), cognitive restructuring + left DLPFC rTMS was associated with enhanced emotion regulation, distress reduction, and increased use of cognitive restructuring compared to sham rTMS.[46]

There is similarly limited support for tDCS as a CBT enhancer. A sham-controlled trial suggests that tDCS does not enhance group CBT for MDD,[47] and a recent (likely underpowered) pilot trial failed to find that tDCS enhanced group CBT for rumination.[48] There are two published RCT protocols investigating tDCS as an add-on of CBT for MDD,[49,50] but the findings have yet to be published.

YOHIMBINE

Yohimbine, an α2-adrenergic receptor antagonist which enhances fear extinction in animals,[51] has promising preliminary support as an enhancer of exposure-based interventions. Yohimbine, relative to placebo, resulted in faster improvement and decreased self-reported, but not clinician-rated, social anxiety and depression during a brief exposure-based treatment for SAD, but only for participants who reported low fear at the end of each exposure.[52] When combined with PE for combat-related PTSD, a single dose of yohimbine resulted in higher arousal during imaginal exposure, greater between-session habituation, and lower arousal in response to trauma cues 1 week later.[53] In addition, yohimbine administration before exposure for claustrophobia was associated with greater reductions in clinical outcomes with large effect sizes.[54] However, yohimbine did not enhance virtual reality exposure for phobia of flying or heights.[55,56]

OTHER AUGMENTATIONS WITH PRELIMINARY DATA
Estradiol

Estrogen has been found to affect fear extinction recall and thus may be an explanatory factor for sex differences in rates of anxiety-related disorders.[57] Specifically, estradiol potentiates activity in the medial PFC, thought to be critical to the extinction of learned fear.[58,59] Administration of exogenous estradiol has therefore been proposed as an adjunctive treatment for fear-based disorders, specifically PTSD.[60] Although preclinical studies are promising,[61] no RCTs comparing CBT + estradiol to CBT alone have been conducted.

Oxytocin

Oxytocin is a neuropeptide that disrupts signals from the amygdala to the autonomic nervous system[62,63] and, therefore, has been proposed as an augmentation strategy for fear-based disorders. Unfortunately, evidence of its utility is lacking. Compared to placebo, intranasal oxytocin improved self-evaluations of performance during exposure for SAD, but these changes did not translate to improved treatment outcomes.[64] In addition, intranasal oxytocin *impeded* treatment response in exposure for arachnophobia compared to a placebo.[65] A pilot trial suggests that intranasal oxytocin may augment PE for PTSD, but observed between-group differences were not significant, likely due to insufficient power.[66] There are two published RCT protocols examining oxytocin + PE for veterans with PTSD,[67,68] but findings have yet to be published.

Methylene Blue

Methylene blue, an autoxidizing agent that enhances fear extinction in animals,[69] has limited support as an add-on for exposure-based interventions. Methylene blue administered after exposure was associated with less claustrophobic fear at follow-up, but only for participants displaying low fear at the end of the extinction trials.[70] For participants with moderate to high fear after exposure, those who received methylene blue evidenced worse outcomes at follow-up than those who received a placebo. In addition, methylene blue combined with a brief daily imaginal exposure intervention did not result in greater reduction in PTSD symptoms than did exposure + placebo or standard PE, but was associated with enhanced evaluator-rated treatment response and quality of life.[71]

Cannabidiol

Cannabidiol (CBD) has also been proposed as a potential CBT augmentation strategy. The human endogenous cannabinoid system is involved in fear extinction,[72] and CBD binds to cannabinoid receptors and may potentiate the endogenous cannabinoid system. In addition, CBD may reduce anxiety by acting as an agonist for serotonin 1A receptors, among other potential pathways whose role in fear extinction is yet unclear.[73] A preclinical study found that CBD enhanced fear extinction among healthy adults,[74] but no differences were found in treatment outcome between treatment-refractory patients with anxiety disorders who received CBD before exposure sessions compared with placebo.[75] Another study examining CBD as an adjunctive treatment for PTSD during PE is currently underway (https://clinicaltrials.gov/study/NCT05132699).

CONSIDERATIONS FOR FUTURE RESEARCH

One topic that merits further inquiry is the use of ketamine, a dissociative drug recently approved to treat treatment-resistant depression, to augment CBT. Ketamine is thought to increase neurogenesis and BDNF levels in the amygdala and hippocampus, which may affect memory reconsolidation and thus be useful in the treatment of PTSD.[76] To date, however, no RCTs have been conducted examining CBT + ketamine versus CBT alone, and the only preliminary evidence of the efficacy of such an approach is in the form of uncontrolled case studies. Relatedly, there is increasing interest in the use of psychedelics, such as psilocybin and lysergic acid diethylamide-25, to potentiate CBT. As this is the topic of another article in this volume, we will not review that literature here.

Future research should investigate the role of real-time functional magnetic resonance imaging neurofeedback (NF) as an adjunct to CBT. NF consists of training participants to upregulate or downregulate activity in a specific brain region based on feedback. For example, patients with depression who received NF targeting the amygdala (which is involved in emotional processing) in response to positive memories showed lower depression severity at post-NF than did depressed patients who received NF targeting a different region (a parietal region that is not involved in emotional processing).[77] In another study, patients with spider phobia who were trained to upregulate DLPFC activity and downregulate insula activity based on NF during symptom provocation (viewing pictures of spiders) demonstrated lower anxiety after treatment than did control patients who did not receive NF.[78] We would suggest, based on this promising preliminary evidence, that adding NF to CBT might help patients make quicker and more targeted clinical gains by providing them with information on how their brains are reacting to their use of therapeutic exercises.

SUMMARY

In this article, we have synthesized the literature on the use of various augmentations of CBT. Although traditional psychopharmacology, such as antidepressant medications, may be of some added benefit, the effects are small when combined with CBT. However, the DCS research conducted over the past 2 decades demonstrates that it is possible to identify and potentiate specific brain mechanisms associated with CBT response. Although the overall effect of DCS is small and results have been mixed, this line of research nevertheless serves as proof of concept that the biological mechanisms of CBT can be potentiated. Ongoing research suggests that exercise, rTMS, and yohimbine are promising, and more research is needed to determine whether and how compounds such as estradiol, methylene blue, and CBD affect the mechanisms of CBT.

CLINICS CARE POINTS

- Traditional pharmacotherapy has only a small Adding traditional pharmacotherapy to CBT yields a small but significant benefit.
- New directions for CBT augmentation include d-cycloserine an, exercise, and non-invasive brain stimulation.
- Other compounds with less research data suggest future directions for inquiry.

DISCLOSURE

Dr D.F. Tolin receives royalties from Guilford Press, John Wiley and Sons, New Harbinger Publications, Oxford University Press, Cambridge University Press, and PsychWire. He is a consultant for Oui Therapeutics and Mindyra LLC. Drs K.A. Lord and K.A. Knowles have no potential conflicts to declare.

REFERENCES

1. Hofmann SG, Smits JA. Cognitive-behavioral therapy for adult anxiety disorders: a meta-analysis of randomized placebo-controlled trials. J Clin Psychiatry 2008; 69(4):621–32.
2. Cuijpers P, Berking M, Andersson G, et al. A meta-analysis of cognitive-behavioural therapy for adult depression, alone and in comparison with other treatments. Can J Psychiatry 2013;58(7):376–85.
3. Loerinc AG, Meuret AE, Twohig MP, et al. Response rates for CBT for anxiety disorders: Need for standardized criteria. Clin Psychol Rev 2015;42:72–82.
4. Cuijpers P, Karyotaki E, Ciharova M, et al. The effects of psychotherapies for depression on response, remission, reliable change, and deterioration: A meta-analysis. Acta Psychiatr Scand 2021;144(3):288–99.
5. Moncrieff J, Kirsch I. Efficacy of antidepressants in adults. BMJ 2005;331(7509): 155–7.
6. Bandelow B, Reitt M, Rover C, et al. Efficacy of treatments for anxiety disorders: a meta-analysis. Int Clin Psychopharmacol 2015;30(4):183–92.
7. Fournier JC, DeRubeis RJ, Hollon SD, et al. Antidepressant drug effects and depression severity: a patient-level meta-analysis. JAMA 2010;303(1):47–53.

8. Tolin DF. Can cognitive behavioral therapy for anxiety and depression be improved with pharmacotherapy? A meta-analysis. Psychiatr Clin North Am 2017;40(4):715–38.

9. Barlow DH, Gorman JM, Shear MK, et al. Cognitive-behavioral therapy, imipramine, or their combination for panic disorder: A randomized controlled trial. JAMA 2000;283(19):2529–36.

10. Marks IM, Swinson RP, Basoglu M, et al. Alprazolam and exposure alone and combined in panic disorder with agoraphobia. A controlled study in London and Toronto. Br J Psychiatry 1993;162:776–87.

11. Quirk GJ, Mueller D. Neural mechanisms of extinction learning and retrieval. Neuropsychopharmacology 2008;33(1):56–72.

12. Falls WA, Miserendino MJ, Davis M. Extinction of fear-potentiated startle: blockade by infusion of an NMDA antagonist into the amygdala. J Neurosci 1992;12(3):854–63.

13. Walker DL, Ressler KJ, Lu KT, et al. Facilitation of conditioned fear extinction by systemic administration or intra-amygdala infusions of D-cycloserine as assessed with fear-potentiated startle in rats. J Neurosci 2002;22(6):2343–51.

14. Guastella AJ, Dadds MR, Lovibond PF, et al. A randomized controlled trial of the effect of D-cycloserine on exposure therapy for spider fear. J Psychiatr Res 2007; 41(6):466–71.

15. Ressler KJ, Rothbaum BO, Tannenbaum L, et al. Cognitive enhancers as adjuncts to psychotherapy: use of D-cycloserine in phobic individuals to facilitate extinction of fear. Arch Gen Psychiatry 2004;61(11):1136–44.

16. Otto MW, Pollack MH, Dowd SM, et al. Randomized trial of d-cycloserine enhancement of cognitive-behavioral therapy for panic disorder. Depress Anxiety 2016;33(8):737–45.

17. Wilhelm S, Buhlmann U, Tolin DF, et al. Augmentation of behavior therapy with D-cycloserine for obsessive-compulsive disorder. Am J Psychiatry 2008;165(3): 335–41 [quiz. 409].

18. Andersson E, Hedman E, Enander J, et al. D-cycloserine vs placebo as adjunct to cognitive behavioral therapy for obsessive-compulsive disorder and interaction with antidepressants: A randomized clinical trial. JAMA Psychiatr 2015; 72(7):659–67.

19. Hofmann SG, Meuret AE, Smits JA, et al. Augmentation of exposure therapy with D-cycloserine for social anxiety disorder. Arch Gen Psychiatry 2006;63(3): 298–304.

20. Tart CD, Handelsman PR, Deboer LB, et al. Augmentation of exposure therapy with post-session administration of D-cycloserine. J Psychiatr Res 2013;47(2): 168–74.

21. Smits JA, Rosenfield D, Otto MW, et al. D-cycloserine enhancement of exposure therapy for social anxiety disorder depends on the success of exposure sessions. J Psychiatr Res 2013;47(10):1455–61.

22. Smits JA, Rosenfield D, Otto MW, et al. D-cycloserine enhancement of fear extinction is specific to successful exposure sessions: evidence from the treatment of height phobia. Biol Psychiatry 2013;73(11):1054–8.

23. Smits JAJ, Pollack MH, Rosenfield D, et al. Dose timing of d-cycloserine to augment exposure therapy for social anxiety disorder: A randomized clinical trial. JAMA Netw Open 2020;3(6):e206777.

24. Mataix-Cols D, Fernandez de la Cruz L, Monzani B, et al. D-cycloserine augmentation of exposure-based cognitive behavior therapy for anxiety, obsessive-

compulsive, and posttraumatic stress disorders: A systematic review and meta-analysis of individual participant data. JAMA Psychiatr 2017;74(5):501–10.

25. Kvam S, Kleppe CL, Nordhus IH, et al. Exercise as a treatment for depression: A meta-analysis. J Affect Disord 2016;202:67–86.

26. Stubbs B, Vancampfort D, Rosenbaum S, et al. An examination of the anxiolytic effects of exercise for people with anxiety and stress-related disorders: A meta-analysis. Psychiatry Res 2017;249:102–8.

27. Kandola A, Vancampfort D, Herring M, et al. Moving to Beat Anxiety: Epidemiology and Therapeutic Issues with Physical Activity for Anxiety. Curr Psychiatry Rep 2018/07/24 2018;20(8):63.

28. Powers MB, Medina JL, Burns S, et al. Exercise Augmentation of Exposure Therapy for PTSD: Rationale and Pilot Efficacy Data. Cognit Behav Ther 2015/07/04 2015;44(4):314–27.

29. Moylan S, Eyre HA, Maes M, et al. Exercising the worry away: How inflammation, oxidative and nitrogen stress mediates the beneficial effect of physical activity on anxiety disorder symptoms and behaviours. Neurosci Biobehav Rev 2013;37(4):573–84.

30. Szuhany KL, Otto MW. Efficacy evaluation of exercise as an augmentation strategy to brief behavioral activation treatment for depression: a randomized pilot trial. Cognit Behav Ther 2020;49(3):228–41.

31. Sabourin BC, Stewart SH, Watt MC, et al. Running as Interoceptive Exposure for Decreasing Anxiety Sensitivity: Replication and Extension. Cognit Behav Ther 2015;44(4):264–74.

32. Meyer JD, Perkins SL, Brower CS, et al. Feasibility of an Exercise and CBT Intervention for Treatment of Depression: A Pilot Randomized Controlled Trial. Clinical Trial. Front Psychiatry 2022;13.

33. Abdollahi A, LeBouthillier DM, Najafi M, et al. Effect of exercise augmentation of cognitive behavioural therapy for the treatment of suicidal ideation and depression. J Affect Disord 2017;219:58–63.

34. Merom D, Phongsavan P, Wagner R, et al. Promoting walking as an adjunct intervention to group cognitive behavioral therapy for anxiety disorders—A pilot group randomized trial. J Anxiety Disord 2008;22(6):959–68.

35. Tatti E, Phillips AL, Paciorek R, et al. Boosting psychological change: Combining non-invasive brain stimulation with psychotherapy. Neurosci Biobehav Rev 2022/11/01/2022;142:104867.

36. Regenold WT, Deng Z-D, Lisanby SH. Noninvasive neuromodulation of the prefrontal cortex in mental health disorders. Neuropsychopharmacology 2022/01/01 2022;47(1):361–72.

37. Duan H, Yan X, Meng S, et al. Effectiveness Evaluation of Repetitive Transcranial Magnetic Stimulation Therapy Combined with Mindfulness-Based Stress Reduction for People with Post-Stroke Depression: A Randomized Controlled Trial. Int J Environ Res Public Health 2023;20(2). https://doi.org/10.3390/ijerph20020930.

38. Carmi L, Tendler A, Bystritsky A, et al. Efficacy and Safety of Deep Transcranial Magnetic Stimulation for Obsessive-Compulsive Disorder: A Prospective Multicenter Randomized Double-Blind Placebo-Controlled Trial. Am J Psychiatry 2019;176(11):931–8.

39. Isserles M, Shalev AY, Roth Y, et al. Effectiveness of deep transcranial magnetic stimulation combined with a brief exposure procedure in post-traumatic stress disorder–a pilot study. Brain Stimul 2013;6(3):377–83.

40. Isserles M, Tendler A, Roth Y, et al. Deep Transcranial Magnetic Stimulation Combined With Brief Exposure for Posttraumatic Stress Disorder: A Prospective Multisite Randomized Trial. Biol Psychiatry 2021;90(10):721–8.

41. Fryml LD, Pelic CG, Acierno R, et al. Exposure Therapy and Simultaneous Repetitive Transcranial Magnetic Stimulation: A Controlled Pilot Trial for the Treatment of Posttraumatic Stress Disorder. J ECT 2019;35(1):53–60.

42. Deppermann S, Vennewald N, Diemer J, et al. Neurobiological and clinical effects of fNIRS-controlled rTMS in patients with panic disorder/agoraphobia during cognitive-behavioural therapy. Neuroimage Clin 2017;16:668–77.

43. Deppermann S, Vennewald N, Diemer J, et al. Does rTMS alter neurocognitive functioning in patients with panic disorder/agoraphobia? An fNIRS-based investigation of prefrontal activation during a cognitive task and its modulation via sham-controlled rTMS. BioMed Res Int 2014;2014:542526.

44. Deppermann S, Notzon S, Kroczek A, et al. Functional co-activation within the prefrontal cortex supports the maintenance of behavioural performance in fear-relevant situations before an iTBS modulated virtual reality challenge in participants with spider phobia. Behav Brain Res 2016;307:208–17.

45. Notzon S, Deppermann S, Fallgatter A, et al. Psychophysiological effects of an iTBS modulated virtual reality challenge including participants with spider phobia. Biol Psychol 2015;112:66–76.

46. Neacsiu AD, Beynel L, Graner JL, et al. Enhancing cognitive restructuring with concurrent fMRI-guided neurostimulation for emotional dysregulation-A randomized controlled trial. J Affect Disord 2022;301:378–89.

47. Aust S, Brakemeier E-L, Spies J, et al. Efficacy of Augmentation of Cognitive Behavioral Therapy With Transcranial Direct Current Stimulation for Depression: A Randomized Clinical Trial. JAMA Psychiatr 2022;79(6):528–37.

48. Horczak P, Wang C, De Witte S, et al. Combining transcranial direct current stimulation with group cognitive behavioral therapy developed to treat rumination: a clinical pilot study. Original Research. Front Neurol 2023;14. https://doi.org/10.3389/fneur.2023.1167029.

49. Carvalho S, Gonçalves ÓF, Brunoni AR, et al. Transcranial Direct Current Stimulation as an Add-on Treatment to Cognitive-Behavior Therapy in First Episode Drug-Naïve Major Depression Patients: The ESAP Study Protocol. Study Protocol. Front Psychiatry 2020. https://doi.org/10.3389/fpsyt.2020.563058.

50. Bajbouj M, Aust S, Spies J, et al. PsychotherapyPlus: augmentation of cognitive behavioral therapy (CBT) with prefrontal transcranial direct current stimulation (tDCS) in major depressive disorder-study design and methodology of a multicenter double-blind randomized placebo-controlled trial. Eur Arch Psychiatry Clin Neurosci 2018;268(8):797–808.

51. Morris RW, Bouton ME. The effect of yohimbine on the extinction of conditioned fear: a role for context. Behav Neurosci 2007;121(3):501–14.

52. Smits JAJ, Rosenfield D, Davis ML, et al. Yohimbine Enhancement of Exposure Therapy for Social Anxiety Disorder: A Randomized Controlled Trial. Biol Psychiatry 2014;75(11):840–6.

53. Tuerk PW, Wangelin BC, Powers MB, et al. Augmenting treatment efficiency in exposure therapy for PTSD: a randomized double-blind placebo-controlled trial of yohimbine HCl. Cognit Behav Ther 2018;47(5):351–71.

54. Powers MB, Smits JAJ, Otto MW, et al. Facilitation of fear extinction in phobic participants with a novel cognitive enhancer: A randomized placebo controlled trial of yohimbine augmentation. J Anxiety Disord 2009;23(3):350–6.

55. Meyerbröker K, Morina N, Emmelkamp PMG. Enhancement of exposure therapy in participants with specific phobia: A randomized controlled trial comparing yohimbine, propranolol and placebo. J Anxiety Disord 2018;57:48–56.
56. Meyerbroeker K, Powers MB, van Stegeren A, et al. Does Yohimbine Hydrochloride Facilitate Fear Extinction in Virtual Reality Treatment of Fear of Flying? A Randomized Placebo-Controlled Trial. Psychother Psychosom 2011;81(1):29–37.
57. Hsu C-MK, Ney LJ, Honan C, et al. Gonadal steroid hormones and emotional memory consolidation: A systematic review and meta-analysis. Neurosci Biobehav Rev 2021;130:529–42.
58. Quirk GJ, Garcia R, Gonzalez-Lima F. Prefrontal mechanisms in extinction of conditioned fear. Biol Psychiatry 2006;60(4):337–43.
59. Milad MR, Quirk GJ. Neurons in medial prefrontal cortex signal memory for fear extinction. Nature 2002;420(6911):70–4.
60. Glover EM, Jovanovic T, Norrholm SD. Estrogen and Extinction of Fear Memories:Implications for Posttraumatic Stress Disorder Treatment. Biol Psychiatry 2015; 78(3):178–85.
61. Graham BM, Milad MR. Blockade of estrogen by hormonal contraceptives impairs fear extinction in female rats and women. Biol Psychiatry 2013;73(4):371–8.
62. Huber D, Veinante P, Stoop R. Vasopressin and oxytocin excite distinct neuronal populations in the central amygdala. Science 2005;308(5719):245–8.
63. Kirsch P, Esslinger C, Chen Q, et al. Oxytocin modulates neural circuitry for social cognition and fear in humans. J Neurosci 2005;25(49):11489–93.
64. Guastella AJ, Howard AL, Dadds MR, et al. A randomized controlled trial of intranasal oxytocin as an adjunct to exposure therapy for social anxiety disorder. Psychoneuroendocrinology 2009;34(6):917–23.
65. Acheson DT, Feifel D, Kamenski M, et al. Intranasal oxytocin administration prior to exposure therapy for arachnophobia impedes treatment response. Depress Anxiety 2015;32(6):400–7.
66. Flanagan JC, Sippel LM, Wahlquist A, et al. Augmenting Prolonged Exposure therapy for PTSD with intranasal oxytocin: A randomized, placebo-controlled pilot trial. J Psychiatr Res 2018;98:64–9.
67. Flanagan JC, Mitchell JM, Baker NL, et al. Enhancing prolonged exposure therapy for PTSD among veterans with oxytocin: Design of a multisite randomized controlled trial. Contemp Clin Trials 2020;95:106074.
68. Back SE, Flanagan JC, Killeen T, et al. COPE and oxytocin for the treatment of co-occurring PTSD and alcohol use disorder: Design and methodology of a randomized controlled trial in U.S. military veterans. Contemp Clin Trials 2023;126: 107084.
69. Wrubel KM, Barrett D, Shumake J, et al. Methylene blue facilitates the extinction of fear in an animal model of susceptibility to learned helplessness. Neurobiol Learn Mem 2007;87(2):209–17.
70. Telch MJ, Bruchey AK, Rosenfield D, et al. Effects of post-session administration of methylene blue on fear extinction and contextual memory in adults with claustrophobia. Am J Psychiatry 2014;171(10):1091–8.
71. Zoellner LA, Telch M, Foa EB, et al. Enhancing extinction learning in posttraumatic stress disorder with brief daily imaginal exposure and methylene blue: A randomized controlled trial. J Clin Psychiatry 2017;78(7):e782–9.
72. Heitland I, Klumpers F, Oosting RS, et al. Failure to extinguish fear and genetic variability in the human cannabinoid receptor 1. Transl Psychiatry 2012;2(9): e162.

73. Lee JLC, Bertoglio LJ, Guimaraes FS, et al. Cannabidiol regulation of emotion and emotional memory processing: relevance for treating anxiety-related and substance abuse disorders. Br J Pharmacol 2017;174(19):3242–56.
74. Das RK, Kamboj SK, Ramadas M, et al. Cannabidiol enhances consolidation of explicit fear extinction in humans. Psychopharmacology (Berl) 2013;226(4): 781–92.
75. Kwee CMB, Baas JMP, van der Flier FE, et al. Cannabidiol enhancement of exposure therapy in treatment refractory patients with social anxiety disorder and panic disorder with agoraphobia: A randomised controlled trial. Eur Neuropsychopharmacol 2022;59:58–67.
76. Duek O, Kelmendi B, Pietrzak RH, et al. Augmenting the Treatment of PTSD with Ketamine—a Review. Current Treatment Options in Psychiatry 2019;6:143–53.
77. Young KD, Siegle GJ, Zotev V, et al. Randomized clinical trial of real-time fMRI amygdala neurofeedback for major depressive disorder: Effects on symptoms and autobiographical memory recall. Am J Psychiatry 2017;174(8):748–55.
78. Zilverstand A, Sorger B, Sarkheil P, et al. fMRI neurofeedback facilitates anxiety regulation in females with spider phobia. Front Behav Neurosci 2015;9:148.

Psychedelics and Evidence-based Psychotherapy
A Systematic Review with Recommendations for Advancing Psychedelic Therapy Research

Lewis Leone, MS[a], Bryan McSpadden, BA[a],
Annamarie DeMarco, BS[b], Lauren Enten, BSA[b], Rachel Kline, BA[b],
Gregory A. Fonzo, PhD[b],*

KEYWORDS

- Psychedelics • Psychedelic-assisted therapy • Evidence-based treatment
- Treatment development

KEY POINTS

- The present systematic review identified substantial variability in the type of psychological intervention provided across clinical trials with psychedelics.
- Observations include a general lack of consistency in psychotherapy type and implementation employed across trials, an inability to disentangle the psychotherapeutic effect as distinct from or in interaction with the drug effect, and no clear optimal psychotherapeutic treatment or framework to complement psychedelic administration.
- Further foundational work is needed to inform understanding of relative contributions of drug and therapy components to clinical efficacy and how to optimally combine psychedelics with psychotherapeutic approaches to maximize therapeutic effects.

INTRODUCTION

Psychedelics, typically referring to serotonergic hallucinogens, belong to a category of substances that primarily exert their profound subjective effects through activation of serotonin (5-HT) 2A receptors.[1] Known as classical psychedelics, these compounds include psilocybin, lysergic acid diethylamide (LSD), mescaline, and N,N-dimethyltryptamine (DMT). Other compounds, which are not classical psychedelics

[a] Department of Psychology, The University of Texas at Austin, Sarah M. and Charles E. Seay Building 108 E. Dean Keeton Street, Mail Stop A8000, Austin, TX 78712, USA; [b] Department of Psychiatry and Behavioral Sciences, Center for Psychedelic Research and Therapy, The University of Texas at Austin Dell Medical School, Health Discovery Building (HDB), 1601 Trinity Street, Building B, Z0600, Austin, TX 78712, USA
* Corresponding author.
E-mail address: gfonzo@austin.utexas.edu

Psychiatr Clin N Am 47 (2024) 367–398
https://doi.org/10.1016/j.psc.2024.02.006
0193-953X/24/© 2024 Elsevier Inc. All rights reserved.

but have been found to produce psychedelic-like effects–such as intensified emotional experience, dissociation, and altered perception–include ketamine, 3,4-methylenedioxymethamphetamine (MDMA), and ibogaine.[1]

Over the past several decades, several clinical trials have demonstrated initial efficacy of psilocybin or MDMA in the treatment of a variety of psychiatric disorders, including major depressive disorder (MDD; eg, see Goodwin and colleagues[2]), posttraumatic stress disorder (PTSD; eg, see Mitchell and colleagues[3]), alcohol-use disorder (AUD; eg, see Bogenschutz and colleagues[4]), and tobacco-use disorder (TUD; eg, Johnson and colleagues[5]). Considering these positive findings, it is increasingly possible that MDMA and/or psilocybin will eventually receive Food and Drug Administration (FDA) approval and become a bona fide psychiatric intervention.

Due to the acute and intense psychological/perceptual effects of psychedelics, the administration and usage of these drugs in research settings has typically incorporated supportive psychological interventions (ketamine has been the primary exception). Moreover, it has been hypothesized that the mechanism of action whereby psychedelics confer therapeutic benefit involves a combination of their pharmacologic effect (ie, mediated at the cellular, neuronal, or circuit-level) and the psychological change facilitated by the phenomenological experience provoked by the compounds.[6] The term psychedelic-assisted therapy (PAT) is a widely used label to describe a treatment involving psychedelic administration combined with a psychological component intended to optimize drug safety and efficacy.

At present, PAT is a broad term without a straightforward definition. Previous reviews[6–9] of the variety of PATs currently utilized in research settings revealed an array of differing approaches. Following Brennan and Belser,[6] these approaches might be usefully divided between "basic support" models and "evidence-based therapy (EBT)-inclusive" models, which are distinguished by the presence or lack of an EBT component that has been established outside of the domain of psychedelic administration. These may include, for instance, acceptance and commitment therapy (ACT) or cognitive behavioral therapy (CBT). All models of PAT generally include 3 components: one or more preparation sessions to provide psychoeducation on psychedelics and prepare the patient for treatment; a dosing session wherein the drug is administered in the presence of one or more trained therapists; and one or more integration sessions during which patients meet with one or more therapists to discuss the content and meaning of their psychedelic experience.[6] Beyond these commonalities, there are prominent differences in how each of these components is implemented in terms of therapist–patient interaction and overall therapeutic framework underlying the psychological treatment component.

The role of psychotherapy (whether primarily facilitating safety or contributing to efficacy) in psychedelic clinical trials remains uncertain. This uncertainty is exacerbated by variability in implementation and the challenge of measuring the specific contributions of the drug, the therapy, and their combination. Nonetheless, there is some evidence that certain psychological elements–for instance, quality of the acute drug experience[10,11] and therapeutic alliance[12]–may contribute to positive outcomes following psychedelic treatment. Furthermore, there are informed clinical and theoretic reasons to suggest that psychotherapy may interact with psychedelic administration to impact clinical outcomes.[6,13,14] As one example, it has been suggested that certain foundational concepts derived from established EBTs—such as the ACT concept of psychological flexibility—are highly relevant to the psychedelic experience and that combining ACT with drug administration may promote beneficial synergistic treatment effects.[13] Other therapeutic techniques used in third-wave CBTs, such as mindfulness and maintaining contact with the present moment, may also be helpful in allowing the participant to optimally navigate the psychedelic experience and any difficult emotional states that may arise therein. Given that the quality of the acute drug experience has been shown, in some cases, to predict more favorable therapeutic responses,[10,11] optimizing the subjective experience of drug effects through psychotherapeutic approaches may be an important factor in improving clinical outcomes. That being said, a comprehensive understanding of the optimal combination of therapy and drug is far from established, and some investigators have argued that there is minimal empirical evidence for any additional benefit conferred by psychotherapy in the context of psychedelic treatment as currently implemented, at least in the case of psilocybin.[15]

Given our nascent understanding of psychedelics and PATs, the current time represents an opportunity for researchers trained in development and validation of psychological treatments to contribute to the improvement and elaboration of methodologies used to incorporate psychedelics into maximally effective treatments for psychiatric disorders.

Toward that end, we provide an up-to-date systematic review and evaluation of the contemporary integration of EBTs with psychedelic compounds in available clinical trials to provide a baseline of where EBT-informed PAT research currently stands, assess next steps for researchers, and provide recommendations for point-of-care clinicians.

METHODS

The authors conducted a systematic review of all psychedelic clinical trials published within the past 20 years, since 2003. This time-period was selected to gather information on modern-day psychedelic medicine while excluding older studies that have historical relevance but are not indicative of the current research landscape. Additional inclusion, search, and data extraction strategies are described in detail later.

Inclusion Criteria

To be eligible for this review, a study must have included a human clinical trial design in one or more well-controlled, standardized medical/academic settings that involved the administration of at least one dose of a psychedelic or psychedelic-like compound (broadly defined, ie, not only limited to serotonergic compounds) for the purpose of treating a mental health-related outcome in a well-defined clinical group and described provision of a psychological intervention component to augment or support therapeutic efficacy or safety. This included studies that examined classical psychedelics (psilocybin, LSD, mescaline, ayahuasca, DMT, 5-MeO DMT) as well as studies involving the administration of MDMA, ketamine, and ibogaine for a clinical condition. To achieve an understanding of the current landscape of PAT, only studies published in the last 20 years were included.

Search Methods

Two databases, PubMed and EMBASE, were each searched on August 2, 2023. Three search strings were used: "psychedelic OR psilocybin OR LSD OR Ayahuasca OR MDMA OR Ketamine OR DMT OR 5-MeO-DMT OR Mescaline OR Ibogaine," "psychedelic-assisted OR LSD-assisted OR psilocybin-assisted OR MDMA-assisted OR Ayahuasca-assisted OR Ketamine-assisted OR DMT-assisted OR 5-MeO-DMT-assisted OR Mescaline-assisted OR Ibogaine-assisted," and "psychedelic-enhanced OR LSD-enhanced OR psilocybin-enhanced OR MDMA-enhanced OR Ayahuasca-enhanced OR Ketamine-enhanced OR DMT-enhanced OR 5-MeO-DMT-enhanced OR Mescaline-enhanced OR Ibogaine-enhanced." A "clinical trial" search filter was used on both PubMed and EMBASE. Furthermore, abbreviations such as LSD and DMT were captured in their unabbreviated form within search results.

Study Selection

A PRISMA flow chart in **Fig. 1** details the study selection process. Following a full search of PubMed and EMBASE, studies were initially screened for eligibility based on title and abstract. Studies which made it past this initial screening phase were then read in their entirety by the first author with the assistance of coauthors to determine eligibility.

Data Extraction

Recorded variables from each study included the following: sample population, sample size, study design, dosage, comparator/control conditions, preparatory session details, dosing-session details, integration session details, PAT model, primary outcome results. These are outlined for each study in **Tables 1** and **2**.

RESULTS

Searches on PubMed and EMBASE resulted in the extraction of 10,323 articles (PubMed = 4,262, EMBASE = 6,061). In total, 5,269 duplicates were removed

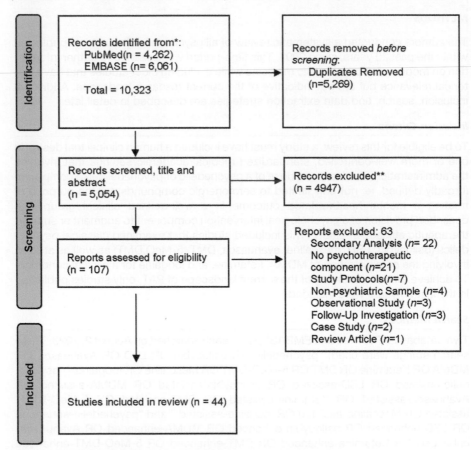

Fig. 1. A PRISMA flow-chart providing details of the study selection process.

Table 1
Summary of Psychedelic Clinical Trials Involving Evidence-based Therapies

Drug	Publication	Design	Disorder and Sample	Doses	Comparator	Prep Support	Dosing Support	Post-dose Support	EBT	Summary of Results
Psilocybin	Johnson et al,[5] 2014	Open label pilot study	Nicotine-dependent smokers (n = 15)	2 dosing sessions optional 3rd dose; Dose 1: 20 mg/70 kg; Dose 2/3: 30 mg/70 kg	None	4 weekly 90 m CBT sessions with 2–3 therapists. "Target Quit Date" set to co-occur with the date of the first psilocybin administration.	At least 1 staff member, music, and eyeshades	1 h meeting 24 h after each dose	CBT	12 of 15 participants (80%) showed 7 day point prevalence abstinence at 6 mo follow-up
Psilocybin	Bogenschutz et al,[19] 2015	Open label pilot	Alcohol dependence (n = 10)	2 dosing sessions Dose 1: 0.3 mg/kg Dose 2: 0.4 mg/kg	None	4 therapy sessions	2 clinicians, music, and eyeshades	4 therapy sessions between the first and second doses, and 4 after second dose	MET	Abstinence did not increase significantly in the first 4 wk of treatment (when participants had not yet received psilocybin), but increased significantly following psilocybin administration
Psilocybin	Anderson et al,[20] 2020	Open label pilot	AIDS-related demoralization (n = 18)	1 dosing session Cohort 1: 0.3 mg/70 kg Cohort 2/3: 0.36 mg/70 kg	None	1 × 90 min individual session; 2 wk of twice weekly 90 min group therapy	2 clinicians, music, and eyeshades	2 h individual therapy with at least 1 therapist following day; then additional twice weekly 90 min group therapy for 2–3 wk	SEGT	Clinically meaningful change in demoralization from baseline to 3 mo follow-up

(continued on next page)

Table 1
(continued)

Drug	Publication	Design	Disorder and Sample	Doses	Comparator	Prep Support	Dosing Support	Post-dose Support	EBT	Summary of Results
Psilocybin	Bogenschutz et al,[4] 2022	Double-blind, placebo-controlled, parallel-arm multi-site RCT	Alcohol dependence (n = 95)	2 dosing sessions Dose 1: 25 mg/70 kg Dose 2: 25–40 mg/70 kg	Diphenhydramine Dose 1: 50 mg Dose 2: 100 mg	4 sessions with 2 therapists	Music and eyeshades	4 sessions between the first and second doses, and 4 after second dose	MET and CBT	Psilocybin group more likely to report no heavy drinking days and reduction in risk level
MDMA	Danforth et al,[23] 2018	Randomized, double-blind placebo-controlled pilot study	Autism w/severe social anxiety disorder (n = 12)	2 dosing sessions Dose 1: 75 mg Dose 1: 125 mg	Lactose	3 preparatory psychotherapy sessions including standardized mindfulness-based therapy adapted from DBT	Supportive psychotherapy	3 non-drug psychotherapy sessions	DBT mindfulness	Improvement in social anxiety from baseline to the primary endpoint was significantly greater for MDMA group compared to the placebo group
MDMA	Monson et al,[24] 2020	Uncontrolled trial	6 Hetero couples (at least 1 partner having PTSD) (n = 12)	2 dosing sessions Dose 1:75 mg Does 2: 100 mg	None	The first 3 sessions of CBCT delivered day before the first MDMA session Sessions 4 and 5 focused delivered in person the morning before MDMA administration	Co-therapists with expertise in MDMA and CBCT, respectively, delivered the therapy sessions	1.5 h session day after MDMA session; additional 4 CBCT sessions in 2 wk following each dosing session	CBCT	There were significant improvements in clinician-assessed, patient-rated, and partner-rated PTSD symptoms
Ketamine	Rodriguez et al,[28] 2016	Open label pilot trial	Obsessive compulsive disorder (n = 10)	1 dosing session 0.5 mg/kg	None	90 min CBT session with therapist	Not reported	10 one hour exposure sessions delivered over 2 weeks	CBT, ERP	At the end of CBT (week 2), 63% of patients demonstrated treatment response (≥35% YBOCS reduction)

| Ketamine | Wilkinson et al,[30] 2017 | Open label trial | Depression (n = 16) | 4 dosing sessions 0.5 mg/kg | None | Not reported | Not reported | CBT 24/48 h following first infusion and provided 2x weekly for 2 wk then 1x weekly for 8 wk (12 total) | CBT | 16 participants initiated the protocol, with 8 (50%) attaining a response to the ketamine and 7 (43.8%) achieving remission during the first 2 wk of protocol. Relapse rate at the end of the CBT course (8 wk following the last ketamine exposure) was 25% (2/8) |
| Ketamine | Dakwar et al,[32] 2019 | Randomized controlled trial | Cocaine dependence (N = 55) | 1 dosing session 0.5 mg/kg | Midazolam 0.025 mg/kg | Received 1 session of MBRP before their ketamine administration on day 2 while hospitalized | Not reported | 3 daily sessions immediately dosing, 5 wk of MBRP administered twice weekly and | MBRP | 48.2% of individuals in the ketamine group maintained abstinence over the last 2 wk of the trial, compared with 10.7% in the midazolam group. Ketamine group was 53% less likely to relapse (compared with the midazolam group) |

(continued on next page)

Table 1
(continued)

Drug	Publication	Design	Disorder and Sample	Doses	Comparator	Prep Support	Dosing Support	Post-dose Support	EBT	Summary of Results
Ketamine	Dakwar et al,[34] 2020	Randomized controlled pilot trial	Alcohol-use disorder (n = 40)	1 dosing session 0.71 mg/kg	Midazolam 0.025 mg/kg	1 session MET before dosing	Not reported	MET session 24 h after dosing session	MET	Ketamine significantly increased the likelihood of abstinence, delayed the time to relapse, and reduced the likelihood of heavy drinking days compared with midazolam
Ketamine	Shiroma et al,[29] 2020	Uncontrolled pilot trial	PTSD (n = 12)	3 dosing sessions 0.5 mg/kg	None	Not reported	Not reported	Up to 10 weekly sessions of prolonged exposure	PE	Scores significantly decreased from baseline to end of treatment in CAPS-5
Ketamine	Wilkinson et al,[31] 2021	Randomized, proof-of-concept trial	Depression (n = 42; n = 28 randomized to CBT or TAU)	6 dosing sessions with TAU or CBT 0.5 mg/kg	None	Not reported	Not reported	CBT was started 24–48 h following the first ketamine infusion, then twice weekly during phase 1 and one per week in phase 2	CBT	28 patients achieved a response from the initial ketamine sessions and were randomized to CBT or TAU. When measured using the MADRS, the effect size at the end of the study was moderate though the group-by-time interaction effect was not significant

Ketamine	Azhari et al,[35] 2021	Controlled proof of concept trial	Cannabis use disorder (n = 8)	1 dosing session or 2 (for non-responders) 0.71 mg/kg; 1.41 mg/kg for non-responders	Not included	MET 1 d before dosing	Mindfulness-based exercises provided throughout	MBRP and MET after first dose before second; MET provided Weeks 3–6		Frequency of cannabis use decreased from baseline to the week following the first infusion, and remained reduced at the end of the study
Ketamine	Grabski et al,[33] 2022	Double blind placebo controlled phase 2 clinical trial	Alcohol use disorder (n = 96)	3 dosing sessions 0.8 mg/kg	Dosing with therapy control (psychoed) Placebo (Saline) with MBRP Placebo (Saline) with therapy control (psychoed)	MBRP or alcohol education (depending on group) 1 d before dosing	Not reported	Ketamine sessions were timed so that the infusion was always preceded by a therapy or alcohol education session and followed by another therapy or alcohol education session about 24 h later	MBRP	Significantly greater number of days abstinent from alcohol in the ketamine group compared with the placebo group at 6 mo follow-up, with the greatest reduction in the ketamine plus therapy group compared with the saline plus education group.

Abbreviations: CBT, cognitive behavioral therapy; DBT, dialectical behavior therapy; ERP, exposure with response prevention; MADRS, Montgomery–Åsberg Depression Rating Scale; MBRP, mindfulness-based relapse prevention; MET, motivational enhancement therapy; PE, prolonged exposure; SEGT, brief supportive expressive group therapy; YBOCS, Yale–Brown Obsessive–Compulsive Scale.

Table 2
Summary of psychedelic clinical trials not involving evidence-based therapies

Drug	Publication	Design	Disorder and Sample	Doses	Comparator	Prep Support	Dosing Support	Post-Dose Support	Therapy Model	Summary of Results
Psilocybin	Moreno et al,[41] 2006	Open label pilot	Obsessive compulsive disorder (n = 9)	Up to 4 dosing sessions 25 μg/kg 100 μg/kg 200 μg/kg 300 μg/kg	None	1 meeting the day before the session	Music and eyeshades	Debrief; Overnight observation in inpatient unit	Therapy model unspecified	Reduction in Y-BOCS scores ranging from 23% to 100%
Psilocybin	Grob et al,[42] 2011	Within-subject, double-blind, placebo-controlled crossover RCT	Cancer-related distress (n = 12)	1 dosing session 0.2 mg/kg	250 mg niacin	Predosing sessions, number of sessions not specified	Music and eyeshades	After session debrief	Therapy model unspecified	Anxiety was significantly reduced at 1 and 3 mo after treatment, significant improvement in mood at 6 mo
Psilocybin	Carhart-Harris et al,[44] 2016	Open label pilot	Depression (n = 12)	2 dosing sessions 10 mg 25 mg	None	4 h session 6 d before first dosing session	Music and eyeshades	Telephone session 1 d after their low-dose; In person support 1 d after their high-dose session	Not specified	Relative to baseline, depressive symptoms were markedly reduced 1 wk and 3 mo after high-dose treatment
Psilocybin	Griffiths et al,[43] 2016	Double-blind, placebo-controlled, parallel-arm multisite RCT	Cancer-related distress (n = 51)	2 dosing sessions 30 mg/70 kg psilocybin	1 mg or 3 mg/70 kg psilocybin	2 or more sessions (mean of ~3 for ~8 h, total)	Music and eyeshades	2+ sessions between 1st and 2nd dosing session (mean of ~3 for ~3 h) and 2+ sessions between 2nd dose and 6 mo follow-up (mean of ~2.5 for ~2.4 h).	Therapy model unspecified	At 6 mo follow-up, response rates for depression were 77%–83% as measured by Hamilton Depression Rating Scale

Drug	Study	Design	Condition	Dosing	Comparator	Preparatory sessions	Supportive	Integration sessions	Therapy model	Outcomes
Psilocybin	Ross et al,[36] 2016	Within-subject, double-blind, placebo-controlled crossover RCT	Cancer-related distress (n = 29)	1 dosing sessions 0.3 mg/kg	250 mg niacin	Three 2 h sessions with therapist dyad for 6 h total over 2–4 wk	Music and eyeshades	3 × 2 h sessions with dyad starting day after dosing	Medication-assisted psychotherapy (mix of existential therapy, CBT, psychodynamic therapy)	Larger reductions in anxiety and depressive symptoms for psilocybin vs niacin
Psilocybin	Carhart-Harris et al,[37] 2021	Double-blind, placebo-controlled parallel arm RCT	Depression (n = 59)	2 dosing sessions 25 mg	2 inactive doses (1 mg) plus 10–20 mg daily escitalopram	3 h preparatory therapeutic session 1 d before first dosing; 1 h preparation session before second dosing session; Accept connect embody model used	Music and eyeshades	1 d post each dosing session + optional additional calls (2 per each session, 1 post treatment)	ACE model	Symptom improvement on QIDS-SR-16. No significant difference between psilocybin and Escitalopram
Psilocybin	Davis et al,[45] 2021	Waitlist-controlled, parallel-arm RCT	Depression (n = 24)	2 dosing sessions Dose 1: 20 mg/70 kg Dose 2: 30 mg/70 kg	Wait list	Preparatory meetings (8 h in total) with 2 session facilitators before the first psilocybin session	Music and eyeshades	Follow-up meetings after psilocybin sessions (2–3 h in total)	Therapy model unspecified	Reduction in HAM-D score for immediate treatment vs waiting list; Rapid reduction in QIDS-SR scores starting 1 d after first dosing session; Benefits largely maintained at 3, 6, and 12 mo post

(continued on next page)

Table 2
(continued)

Drug	Publication	Design	Disorder and Sample	Doses	Comparator	Prep Support	Dosing Support	Post-Dose Support	Therapy Model	Summary of Results
Psilocybin	Goodwin et al,[2] 2022	Double-blind parallel arm RCT	Depression (n = 233)	1 dosing session 25 mg or 10 mg	1 mg psilocybin	3 d of meetings with a therapist during a period of 3–6 wk before the psilocybin session	Music, eyeshades	2 integration sessions at 1 d and 1 wk after	PCT-informed model	Psilocybin at a single dose of 25 mg, but not 10 mg, reduced MADRS scores significantly more than a 1-mg dose over a period of 3 wk but was associated with adverse effect
Psilocybin	Schneier et al,[39] 2023	Open label pilot study	Body dysmorphic disorder (n = 12)	1 dosing session 25 mg	None	4 weekly psychoeducation session w/ relaxation techniques	General psych support from 2 therapists who gave prep, eye shades, music	1 d post admin and 1 wk post admin for debriefing and support processing experience	PCT-informed model	BDD severity significantly lowered with a large effect size across 12 wk of monitoring. 7/12 participants had a greater or equal to 30% decrease in BDD symptoms at every follow up over 12 wk
Psilocybin	Shnayder et al,[46] 2023	Phase II open label clinical trial	Depression in cancer patients (n = 30)	1 dosing session 25 mg	None	Visit 1: 2 h with therapist for coping strategies and psychoeducation. Visit 2 (1 d before dosing): 75 min group psychoeducation and 45 min 1 on 1 w/ therapist to address concerns	Active listening and presence, non-directive support, eye shades, music	75 min single therapy session and 45 min group therapy on both the day after dosing and 1 week after dosing	Therapy model unspecified	Positive change in psycho-social-spiritual well-being. These effects were apparent 1 day after psilocybin treatment and were sustained up to the last study interval at 8 wk

Drug	Study	Design	Population	Dosing	Placebo	Preparatory	Adjuncts	Integration	Therapy model	Outcome (Depression)
Psilocybin	Sloshower et al,[64] 2023	Exploratory placebo-controlled, within-subject, fixed-order study	Depression (n = 19)	1 dosing session 0.3 mg/kg	Microcrystalline cellulose in an dentical capsule	2 h long preparatory psychotherapy/psychoeducation session preceded each dosing session	Music and eyeshades	Two 1 h long debriefing/integration psychotherapy sessions were conducted 1 d and 1 week after each dosing session. Following collection of the final primary outcome measures at week 6, participants had 2 additional integration sessions to help sustain any initial clinical improvements	ACT-informed model	Depression (HAM-D) significantly improved following both placebo and psilocybin with no significant difference in the degree of change between the two conditions
Psilocybin	von Rotz et al,[47] 2023	Double-blind parallel arm RCT	Depression (n = 52)	1 dosing session 0.215 mg/kg	Inactive placebo	2 preparatory sessions 4-6 d and 1 d before psilocybin administration, 1 h each	Music	Three 1 h visits 2 d, 8 d, and 14 d after the intervention	Therapy model unspecified	Psilocybin group showed significantly larger decrease in MADRS scores as compared to the placebo group 14 d after the intervention

(continued on next page)

Table 2
(continued)

Drug	Publication	Design	Disorder and Sample	Doses	Comparator	Prep Support	Dosing Support	Post-Dose Support	Therapy Model	Summary of Results
Psilocybin	Goodwin et al,[38] 2023	Phase II, exploratory open-label study	Depression (n = 19)	1 dosing session 25 mg	None	3 sessions, during which the therapist built trust with the participant, explained the trial design and procedures, provided psychoeducation, and helped to prepare the participant for the psilocybin experience. The final preparation session took place the day before administration	Eyeshades and music	Integration session with their lead therapist who encouraged them to derive their own solutions and insights from the psilocybin experience	PCT-informed model	At week 3, mean change from baseline in MADRS total score was −14.9… Both response and remission were evident in 8 (42.1%) participants
MDMA	Bouso et al,[53] 2008	Double-blind, ascending-dose study, randomized and placebo-controlled	PTSD (N = 6)	1 dosing session 50–75 mg, depending on group	Placebo	3 psychotherapy nondrug session 90 min long	Music, minimal therapeutic discussion	3 psychotherapy nondrug session 90 min long	MDMA-assisted psychotherapy	Low doses of MDMA administered as an adjunct to psychotherapy were found to be safe for the 6 subjects with chronic PTSD treated in this clinical trial and there were promising signs of efficacy and reduced PTSD symptomatology

MDMA	Mithoefer et al,[49] 2011	Randomized controlled pilot study	PTSD (n = 20)	2 dosing sessions 125 mg + optional supplemental dose of 62.5 mg MDMA	Lactose	Two 90 min introductory sessions within 6 wk before the first experimental session to prepare them for the structure of the sessions, the approach to therapy and possible effects of MDMA	Psychological support; option for eyeshades and music	At least 8 integration sessions, and three more were scheduled during the month following each experimental session. Additional integration sessions were permitted if needed	MDMA-assisted psychotherapy	Decrease in CAPS scores from baseline was significantly greater for the group that received MDMA than for the placebo group at all 3 time points after baseline
MDMA	Oehen et al,[52] 2013	Randomized, double-blind, active placebo-controlled	PTSD (n = 12)	3 dosing sessions 125 mg, plus 62.5 mg supplemental dose	3 low dose dosing sessions 25 mg plus 12.5 mg supplemental dose	Two preparatory sessions, aimed at establishing a therapeutic alliance and preparing subjects for the MDMA experience, preceded the first MDMA session of the study	Focused body work, music, hand holding when consented; one male and one female therapist present the whole time	Non-drug psychotherapy session the morning after dosing, followed by 2 sessions that were 1 week apart; therapists contacted daily for a week following	MDMA-assisted psychotherapy	Did not see statistically significant reductions in CAPS scores ($P=.066$), although there was clinically and statistically significant self-reported (PDS) improvement
MDMA	Mithoefer et al,[48] 2018	Randomized, double-blind, dose-response to open-label crossover	PTSD (n = 26)	2 dosing sessions 75 mg 125 mg	2 low-dose dosing sessions 30 mg	Three 90 min preparatory sessions	Manualized MDMA-assisted psychotherapy with a male or female co-therapy team	Overnight stay onsite, 7 d of telephone contact, 13 and three 90 min psychotherapy sessions aimed at integrating the experience	MDMA-assisted psychotherapy	Participants receiving larger doses (75 mg, 125 mg) had significantly greater decreases in PTSD symptom severity than the 30 mg group

(continued on next page)

Table 2
(continued)

Drug	Publication	Design	Disorder and Sample	Doses	Comparator	Prep Support	Dosing Support	Post-Dose Support	Therapy Model	Summary of Results
MDMA	Ot'alora G et al,[51] 2018	Double-blind, dose response; one open-label session	PTSD (n = 28)	2 dosing sessions 100 mg, 125 mg	2 low-dose dosing sessions 40 mg	Three 90 min preparatory sessions	Eyeshades, headphones with instrumental music, an attendant	Integration sessions after first dosing session (90 min); second and third were before the second dosing session (approx. weekly). There were also daily 15–60 min phone calls that occurred for 7 d following each session	MDMA-assisted psychotherapy	PTSD symptoms remained lower than baseline at 12 mo follow-up
MDMA	Wolfson et al,[54] 2020	Double-blinded, randomized, placebo-controlled design with an open-label crossover	Anxiety in people with a life-threatening illness (n = 18)	2 dosing sessions 125 mg followed by an optional supplemental dose of 62.5 mg	125 mg lactose	Three 90 min preparatory sessions	Nondirective therapy throughout the 8-h sessions	Integration sessions 1 day after dosing + two additional integration therapy sessions 1 month later	MDMA-assisted psychotherapy	Mean change in trait anxiety score was greater for the MDMA group, but differences were not statistically significant
MDMA	Jardim et al,[50] 2021	Open label clinical trial	PTSD (n = 3)	3 dosing sessions 112.5 mg 187.5 mg (sessions 2 and 3)	None	Two 1 h psychotherapy sessions including some elements of motivational interviewing and "third wave" cognitive behavioral approaches	MDMA-assisted psychotherapy	3 integration sessions within a month following all 3 MDMA-AP sessions (9 total)	MDMA-assisted psychotherapy	Reductions in CAPS scores for all participants with a large effect size but not statistically significant

MDMA	Mitchell et al,[3] 2021	Randomized, double-blind, placebo-controlled	PTSD (n = 90)	3 dosing sessions 80 mg followed by a supplemental half-dose of 40 mg 120 mg was followed by a supplemental half-dose of 60 mg (sessions 2 and 3)	Nct specified	Three 90 min preparatory sessions of therapy with a two-person therapist team in preparation for experimental sessions	MDMA-assisted psychotherapy	9 integration sessions MDMA-assisted psychotherapy model	MDMA-assisted psychotherapy	MDMA was found to induce significant and robust attenuation in CAPS-5 score compared with placebo
MDMA	Sessa et al,[55] 2021	Open-label, within-subjects proof of concept	Alcohol-use disorder (n = 14)	2 dosing sessions 125 mg MDMA, followed 2 hours later by a booster dose of 62.5 mg MDMA	None	21 h psychotherapy sessions of motivational interviewing and "third wave" cognitive behavioral approaches	MDMA-assisted psychotherapy	2 sessions total the morning after each drug-assisted session; telephoned daily for 6 days to assess changes to mood, suicidal risk factors and quality of sleep	MDMA-assisted psychotherapy	Average units of alcohol consumption by participants was 18.7 units per week compared to 130.6 units per week before the detox
Ketamine	Krupitsky et al,[56] 2007	Randomized controlled trial	Heroin dependence (n = 59)	3 dosing sessions 2.0 mg/kg	1 dosing session only	5 h of psychoeducation before the first session and One hour of addiction counseling was provided before the second and third ketamine sessions	Music	5 h psychotherapy after the first ketamine session. Participants in the multiple ketamine session group also received an additional hour of psychotherapy (ie, integration) after each session	Ketamine-assisted psychotherapy	At 1 y follow-up, survival analysis demonstrated a significantly higher rate of abstinence in the multiple ketamine dosing group. No differences between groups were found in depression, anxiety, craving for heroin, or their understanding of the meaning of their lives

(continued on next page)

Table 2
(continued)

Drug	Publication	Design	Disorder and Sample	Doses	Comparator	Prep Support	Dosing Support	Post-Dose Support	Therapy Model	Summary of Results
Ketamine	Pradhan et al,[57] 2018	Pilot randomized controlled trial	PTSD (n = 20)	1 dosing session 0.5 mg/kg	Normal saline	Not reported	Therapeutic support using TIMBER model	Therapeutic support using TIMBER model: 12 sessions total (1st during infusion); 3 mini sessions on infusion, 2nd day post, and 8th day; 9 full 45 min sessions 1x weekly	Trauma interventions using mindfulness-based extinction and reconsolidation (TIMBER)	Duration of treatment response longer for ketamine arm of treatment
Ketamine	Price et al,[58] 2022	Randomized double-blind, parallel-arm trial	Depression (n = 154)	1 dosing session 0.5 mg/kg	Saline + ASAT ketamine + Sham ASAT	Not reported	Not reported	Computer-based automated self-association training 1 d post infusion: 8 sessions, 2x daily, starting 1 d post dose	Automated self-association training	Ketamine significantly reduced depression scores at 24 h post infusion
Ayahuasca	Palhano-Fontes et al,[59] 2019	Parallel-arm, double-blind, randomized, placebo-controlled trial	Depression (n = 29)	1 dosing session On average Ayahuasca contained 0.36 ± 0.01 mg/mL of N, N-DMT, 1.86 ± 0.11 mg/mL of harmine, 0.24 ± 0.03 mg/mL of harmaline, and 1.20 ± 0.05 mg/mL	Water, yeast, citric acid, zinc sulfate and caramel colorant	Not reported	2 investigators in room offering "support when needed" participants guided to remain quiet, with their eyes closed, while focusing on their body, thoughts, and emotions. They were also allowed to listen to a predefined music playlist	Unspecified support as part of 1 wk inpatient stay for 4 patients presenting in a delicate condition post dosing	Therapy model not specified	Patients treated with ayahuasca showed significantly reduced severity when compared with patients treated with placebo (MADRS-D scores)

Ayahuasca	Dos Santos et al,[60] 2021	Pilot, proof-of-concept, randomized, placebo-controlled trial	Social anxiety disorder (n = 17)	1 dosing session 2 mL/kg	Mineral water (500 mL), glycerin 5% (E422); propylene glycol 5% (E1520); and methylparaben 0.1% (E218)	Creation of trust with the volunteers before the experiment	Nondirective, supportive approach during drug sessions	Not reported	Therapy model unspecified	Compared with placebo, ayahuasca significantly improved self-statements during public speaking scale) and increased somatic symptoms (bodily symptoms scale)
LSD	Gasser et al,[61] 2014	Double-blind randomized placebo controlled clinical trial	Anxiety associated with life-threatening disease (n = 12)	2 dosing sessions 200 μg	20 μg of LSD	2 psychotherapy prep sessions, using "set" guidance	2 therapists, music, LSD-assisted psychotherapy 1/3 brief conversation, 2/3 inner exploration	3 × 60–90 min psychotherapy sessions after each dosing session	Therapy model unspecified	State and trait anxiety significantly reduced
LSD	Holze et al,[62] 2023	Double-blind, placebo-controlled, 2-period, random-order, crossover design	Anxiety associated with life-threatening disease (n = 42)	2 dosing sessions 200 μg	Ethanol	One 1 h psychotherapy session at baseline	Music, eyeshades, therapists	Integration sessions (number of hours not reported)	Therapy model unspecified	SD treatment resulted in significant reductions of state-trait anxiety inventory–global scores up to 16 wk after treatment
DMT	D'Souza et al,[63] 2022	Open-label, fixed-order, dose-escalation	Depression (n = 7)	2 dosing sessions 0.1 mg/kg followed by a 0.3 mg/kg dose of DMT	None	Informational and mood discussion with psychiatrist	Therapist basic support	Post-session phone calls and additional meetings with therapists	Therapy model unspecified	HAMD-17 scores decreased significantly compared to baseline in MDD participants the day after receiving 0.3 mg/kg DMT

Abbreviations: CAPS, clinician-administered PTSD scale for DSM-5; CBT, cognitive behavioral therapy; HAM-D, Hamilton depression rating scale; MADRS, Montgomery–Aasberg depression rating scale; MDD, major depressive disorder; MET, motivational enhancement therapy; PCT, perceptual control theory; PDS, posttraumatic diagnostic scale; QIDS-SR, Quick Inventory of Depressive Symptoms Self-Report; RCT, randomized controlled trial; Y-BOCS, Yale-Brown Obsessive Compulsive Scale.

resulting in 5,054 studies. Of these studies, 4,947 abstracts were screened out of eligibility based on abstracts. From here, 107 studies were read thoroughly to assess for inclusion. Of these 107 studies, 63 were excluded based on inclusion criteria, leaving 44 studies eligible for review.

Psychedelic Clinical Trials Incorporating Evidence-based Therapies

For the purposes of this review, psychedelic clinical trials incorporating an EBT component are recognized specifically as trials that unambiguously included the administration of a full or partial course of a treatment that has demonstrated therapeutic efficacy outside of the domain of psychedelic administration. An outline of the reviewed trials included in this category is detailed later. Additional information regarding dosage, control conditions, and results can be found in **Table 1**.

Psilocybin

Four out of 17 clinical trials (23.5%) involving the administration of psilocybin for a psychiatric disorder indicated the use of an EBT in the trial. These treatments include CBT, motivational enhancement therapy (MET), and brief supportive expressive group therapy (SEGT), each which have displayed efficacy outside the context of psychedelics.[16–18] In one open label pilot study examining the use of psilocybin for 15 smokers with TUD, participants received 4 weekly sessions of CBT for smoking cessation, with a "target quit date," set to co-occur with the date of the first psilocybin administration.[5] In this trial, 12 of 15 participants (80%) showed 7 day point prevalence abstinence at 6 month follow-up. In another open label pilot trial investigating psilocybin-assisted treatment of AUD, 10 participants received 12 psychotherapy sessions, 7 of which included a structured motivational interviewing approach, MET.[19] Abstinence increased significantly following psilocybin administration. A follow-up double-blind, placebo-controlled, parallel-arm multisite randomized controlled trial (RCT) of psilocybin versus diphenhydramine (an active placebo) for 95 participants with AUD included 12 psychotherapy sessions incorporating both CBT and MET therapeutic techniques.[4] By the end of the trial, the psilocybin group demonstrated significantly greater reductions in past-month heavy drinking days. In another open-label pilot study, 18 elderly male adults whom were long-term survivors of acquired immune deficiency syndrome (AIDS) experiencing moderate-to-severe demoralization, a form of existential suffering characterized by poor coping, helplessness, hopelessness, and loss of meaning, underwent 12 to 15 hours of group psychotherapy, which featured a modified administration of brief SEGT prior to and after psilocybin dosing.[20] A clinically meaningful change in demoralization from baseline to 3 month follow-up was observed in this study. No psilocybin trials isolated the specific effect of EBT components through incorporation of psychotherapeutic comparator conditions or drug-only conditions compared to drug-plus psychotherapy.

3,4-Methylenedioxymethamphetamine

Two of 11 (18.2%) of MDMA studies utilized an existing EBT psychological component, including dialectical behavioral therapy (DBT) and cognitive behavioral conjoint therapy (CBCT), which have displayed efficacy outside of the context of psychedelic administration.[21,22] In one study, 12 autistic adults with social anxiety received mindfulness-based therapy adapted directly from DBT in combination with MDMA or placebo in a randomized placebo-controlled study.[23] Improvement in social anxiety from baseline to the endpoint was significantly greater for the MDMA group compared to the placebo group. A separate open-label trial investigated the use of MDMA in couples therapy wherein at least one partner had a PTSD diagnosis.[24] Six heterosexual couples (N = 12) in this trial underwent 15 sessions of CBCT, an EBT which includes psychoeducation about trauma and relationships and therapeutic techniques aimed at increasing relational safety, improving communication skills, and restructuring problematic trauma-related and relationship cognitions. Significant improvements in clinician-assessed, patient-rated, and partner-rated PTSD symptoms were observed in this study. No MDMA trials isolated the specific effect of EBT components through incorporation of psychotherapeutic comparator conditions or drug-only conditions compared to drug-plus psychotherapy.

Ketamine

Eight of 11 (72.7%) reviewed ketamine trials incorporated an EBT. EBTs included exposure with response prevention (ERP), prolonged exposure (PE), mindfulness-based relapse prevention (MBRP), CBT, and MET, which have each demonstrated therapeutic efficacy outside the context of psychedelics.[16,17,25–27] Two open-label trials combined ketamine with exposure-based treatment, including a trial of ERP and CBT for OCD (n = 10),[28] and a trial utilizing PE for PTSD (n = 12).[29] Statistically significant symptom improvements were observed in each of these trials. Two additional trials investigated the combination of CBT and ketamine, and examined how follow-up CBT sessions might sustain postdosing effects.[30,31] In the first of these trials, which featured an open-label design and 16 participants with depression, 8 participants demonstrated a clinically significant response to ketamine, and 7 achieved symptom remission during the first 2 weeks. In a randomized proof-of-concept follow-up trial with 42 participants with depression, 28 patients demonstrated symptom response following initial ketamine sessions and were randomized to CBT or treatment as usual (TAU). Results indicated greater sustained improvement in the CBT group. Two additional RCTs combined ketamine administration with an EBT for AUD.[32,33] The first of these trials investigated ketamine compared to midazolam in 40 participants undergoing a 5 week outpatient regimen of MET and found that ketamine significantly increased the likelihood of abstinence, delayed the time to relapse, and reduced the likelihood of heavy drinking days compared with midazolam.[32] The second of these trials compared ketamine versus saline placebo in 96 participants and featured a 4 arm design including the following treatment conditions: (1) ketamine-plus MBRP, (2) saline-plus MBRP, (3) ketamine-plus psychoeducation, or (2) saline infusion-plus psychoeducation.[33] This trial is unique in that it incorporates design elements that allow for the evaluation of the specific effects of therapy versus a psychoeducation control condition, although it was not adequately powered to assess drug and therapy interaction. Researchers found that ketamine increased the number of days abstinent from alcohol at 3 and 6 months when compared to saline placebo, pooled across therapy conditions. The ketamine-plus MBRP group displayed more days abstinent and lower odds of relapse than the ketamine-plus psychoeducation group; however, this difference did not reach statistical significance. Another RCT combined MBRP with ketamine versus midazolam for cocaine dependence (n = 55), and observed that 48.2% of individuals in the ketamine group maintained abstinence over the last 2 weeks of the trial, compared with 10.7% in the midazolam group.[34] Finally, another open label trial combined both MET and MBRP with ketamine to treat cannabis use disorder (n = 8).[35] Frequency of cannabis use decreased from baseline to the week following the first infusion and remained reduced at the end of the study. Notably, the evidence base for EBT combinations with ketamine is unique among the broader PAT literature in that at least one trial attempted to differentiate the specific impact of an EBT combined with ketamine through comparison to ketamine with psychoeducation,[33] while another aimed to isolate the specific benefits of CBT (vs TAU) in the weeks following dosing to sustain treatment effects for ketamine responders.[31]

Other compounds

No reviewed trials of LSD, ayahuasca, DMT, 5-MeO DMT, or mescaline included the use of an EBT component.

Psychedelic Clinical Trials Not Incorporating EBTs

This category of clinical trials report no incorporation of an EBT developed outside of the context of psychedelic administration. This is inclusive of trials that describe a specific model of PAT (such as MDMA-assisted psychotherapy), trials that incorporate an eclectic mix of psychological interventions from multiple sources without any prior research or evidence base validating the combinations, and trials that do not make any reference to a specific therapeutic model, such as those that only describe basic support conditions. An outline of trials included in this category as differentiated by drug is detailed later. Additional information regarding dosage, control conditions, and results can be found in **Table 2**.

Psilocybin

Three of 17 psilocybin clinical trials did not incorporate a specific EBT (76.5%). Of these trials, 6 of 13 (46.2%) specified a specific support model. These specific models include the medication-assisted psychotherapy (MAP) model, the accept, connect, embody (ACE) model, the Perceptual Control Theory (PCT) model, and an unnamed model that utilizes certain components of ACT. One RCT (n = 29) utilized the MAP model in conjunction with psilocybin (vs niacin) dosing sessions in patients with anxiety and depression associated with life-threatening cancer.[36] In this study, larger reductions in anxiety and depressive symptoms were observed for the psilocybin versus niacin arms. The authors described that psychotherapeutic support in MAP involved a mix of elements drawn from CBT, existentially oriented therapy, and psychodynamic therapy. Another RCT (n = 59) applied elements of the ACE model while comparing psilocybin versus escitalopram (a common antidepressant) for MDD.[37] Participants in this study demonstrated roughly equivalent symptom improvement across arms, and there was no statistically significant difference between psilocybin and escitalopram groups on the primary outcome. The ACE model, though not empirically validated as a standalone treatment, draws heavily on theories of psychological flexibility and shares some similarities with ACT. In addition, several other trials specified the use of a psychological training program for psilocybin therapy that draws heavily from a model known as PCT, a framework where psychological health is considered to represent a homeostatic balance among various biological, psychological, and social variables, which are explored and evaluated through perceptual feedback.[2,38,39] The largest of these trials was a double-blind parallel arm RCT of 3 different psilocybin doses (n = 233), which observed that psilocybin at a single dose of 25 mg, but not 10 mg, reduced symptoms of depression significantly more than a 1 mg dose over a period of 3 weeks.[2] In addition, another RCT (n = 19), which utilized an unnamed model that draws heavily from principles of ACT to treat MDD, observed a significant reduction in depression symptoms in both the treatment and control groups, however the differences in symptom reduction between the two groups of this exploratory study did not reach statistical significance.[40] The remaining trials did not specify a specific therapeutic model, but all included some level of psychological support in the form of preparatory psychoeducation and rapport building, therapeutic presence during dosing sessions, and integration of experience through meetings with therapists in the day or days following treatment.[41–47] No psilocybin trials isolated the specific effect of the psychotherapeutic component through comparison with a drug-only condition.

3,4-Methylenedioxymethamphetamine

Nine of 11 (81.8%) MDMA trials did not report the use of a specific EBT. Each of these MDMA trials incorporated an MDMA-assisted therapy model (MDMA-AT), which has evidential support for the treatment of PTSD only in the context of MDMA trials.[3,48–53] MDMA-AT is a manualized therapy employing a nondirective approach that aims to allow patients to revisit traumatic memories along with related emotions and behavioral patterns. It was developed specifically to pair with the effects of MDMA—such as increased interpersonal trust and reduced fear—as an adjunctive PTSD treatment. The largest study incorporating this therapy modality adopted an RCT design and included 90 participants with PTSD.[3] In this study, MDMA versus placebo was found to induce significant and robust attenuation in PTSD symptoms. Of the remaining 8 studies, 3 others adopted an RCT design,[49,52,53] 3 adopted an RCT design followed by an open-label crossover,[48,51,54] and 2 adopted an open-label design.[50,55] Of these trials, one RCT encompassing only 6 individuals with PTSD was ended prematurely due to political pressures in 2008,[53] while another pilot RCT including 20 participants with PTSD reported significant decreases in PTSD symptoms when compared with inactive placebo.[49] Moreover, a pilot RCT including 12 participants with PTSD observed significant decreases in self-reported PTSD symptoms when MDMA administration was compared to active placebo (low-dose MDMA).[52] Of the 3 studies employing an RCT with subsequent open-label treatment, one observed that MDMA conferred significant decreases in PTSD symptoms in 26 participants when compared to low-dose MDMA.[48] Another study reported the same positive outcome in 28 participants, but results only reached significance in the per-protocol set and not the intent-to-treat set.[51] A third randomized open-label crossover trial—a pilot study investigating MDMA for anxiety associated with life-threatening illness—observed a greater decrease in anxiety in the MDMA group in comparison to inactive placebo, but these results did not reach statistical significance.[54] Of the 2 purely open-label trials, neither observed statistically significant results, but did find that MDMA treatment reduced symptoms and was well tolerated in individuals with PTSD[50] and AUD.[55] No MDMA trials isolated the specific effect of the psychotherapeutic component through comparison with a drug-only condition.

Ketamine

Three of 11 (27.3%) ketamine trials that reported the use of psychosocial components did not report the use of a specific EBT. One RCT investigating the use of 1 versus 3 ketamine doses for heroin dependence in 59 participants described the administration of "ketamine-assisted psychotherapy" and included reference to a preparatory, dosing session, and integrative psychological support.[56] At 1 year follow-up, there was a significantly higher rate of abstinence in those receiving multiple doses. Another pilot RCT outlined the use of a specific model known as trauma interventions using mindfulness-based extinction and reconsolidation (TIMBER), for the treatment of 20 participants with PTSD.[57] TIMBER draws heavily from EBTs such as mindfulness-based cognitive therapy. This study found that the duration of treatment response was longer for the ketamine versus inactive placebo (saline) group. Furthermore, a randomized, double-blind parallel-arm trial examined an active versus sham novel automated intervention called automated self-association training (ASAT), a cognitive training intervention meant to target negative self-evaluation, in combination with ketamine versus saline treatment in 152 individuals with treatment-resistant depression.[58] This study employed 3 cells of a full 2 × 2 factorial, eschewing the saline plus sham ASAT condition. In this study, ketamine treatment was observed to significantly reduce depression scores at 24 hours post-infusion, and the magnitude of benefit was more substantial in the ketamine-plus active ASAT versus saline-plus active ASAT group and longer lasting in the ketamine-plus active ASAT versus ketamine-plus sham ASAT group. Though not incorporating a psychotherapeutic component, this trial is notable for being only one of 2 reviewed studies (the other being an EBT-inclusive ketamine study)[33] that demonstrated evidence of a probable interaction effect between drug and psychological intervention. Trials that did not include any description of a psychotherapeutic component were assumed to use an "infusion-only" model of ketamine administration and therefore were not eligible for this review. No ketamine trials in this group isolated the specific effect of a psychotherapeutic component through comparison with a drug-only condition.

Ayahuasca
Two of 2 (100%) ayahuasca trials did not incorporate the use of an EBT. Each of these trials included some level of psychological support but did not include reference to any specific psychotherapeutic modality or model.[59,60] Both trials utilized a randomized placebo-controlled design and observed symptom improvement in individuals with depression and social anxiety disorder, respectively. There was no comparison of different psychotherapeutic models or an ayahuasca with no psychological support comparator condition.

Lysergic acid diethylamide
Two of 2 (100%) LSD trials did not incorporate EBTs into treatment, but did include some degree of training for therapists to aid in talk therapy for which the details were not fully described.[61,62] The first of these trials featured a dose-comparison RCT design (200 mcg vs 20 mcg of LSD) followed by an open-label crossover to the high-dose condition for the treatment of anxiety associated with life-threatening disease in 12 participants.[61] Following treatment, investigators observed a larger reduction in both state and trait anxiety in the high versus low LSD dose conditions. The more recent trial featured a double-blind, 2 period, random-order, crossover design investigating LSD versus placebo for anxiety associated with life-threatening disease in 42 participants.[62] This trial also observed significantly larger reductions in state and trait anxiety for the blinded LSD versus placebo first period portion. No LSD trials isolated the specific effect of the psychotherapeutic component through comparison with a drug-only condition.

N,N-Dimethyltryptamine
One of 1 trial (100%) utilized DMT for clinical treatment and did not incorporate an EBT. Rather, this study utilized a nondirective and supportive approach in an open label, fixed order dose escalation trial investigating the administration of DMT in both healthy volunteers and individuals with MDD.[63] In this trial, depression symptoms decreased significantly compared to baseline in MDD participants 1 day after the DMT dosing session.

Other compounds
No clinical trials investigating the use of 5-MeO-DMT, mescaline, or ibogaine met our review search criteria.

DISCUSSION

The present review identified substantial variability in the type of psychological intervention provided across clinical trials with psychedelics. These can be categorized as (1) trials that combine psychedelics with a modified form of an existing EBT; (2) trials that use a treatment model developed specifically for psychedelic therapies (such as MDMA-AT and ACE); and trials that provide psychological interventions directed exclusively toward safety and rapport-focused psychological support. Taken together, the evidence base is extremely heterogeneous regarding the content and implementation of psychological interventions in currently published clinical trials of psychedelic compounds. This is further compounded by incomplete reporting of how these components were designed and delivered, which limits inferences on quality and fidelity. Finally, there has been little effort devoted toward disentangling therapeutic effects of the drug and therapy components or their potential interactive effects. Therefore, we propose that knowledge and optimization of the psychological intervention components of PATs can be substantially enhanced through (1) rigorous testing of the efficacy of the psychological components alone (ie, apart from expectancy effects related to the administration of a drug or placebo) and in combination with drug administration; (2) careful experimental design that can tease apart the main and interactive effects of the drug and psychological components in PATs; and (3) head-to-head testing of different psychological intervention components combined with psychedelic compounds in comparative efficacy trials and in trials designed to establish differential mechanisms of change alone and in interaction with drug administration.

The current evidence base is insufficient to identify the optimal psychological interventions to be administered alongside psychedelics for any clinical indication. It remains an open question how to best integrate psychological interventions within the context of psychedelic therapies. While EBTs have the advantage of empirical support for efficacy in specific indications outside the context of psychedelic administration, it remains an assumption that they translate well to bolstering or enhancing the putative therapeutic effects of psychedelic administration in these indications. It is important to note that combining EBTs with psychedelic administration does not make the treatment approach tantamount or superior to provision of the EBT alone—the combination must first undergo rigorous research and evidence—accumulation to earn the EBT title, and comparative efficacy trials are necessary to support the superiority of one psychological treatment approach to another.

Importantly, treatment development of this kind should carefully consider psychological mechanisms of change in psychotherapy. For a combined EBT and psychedelic approach, for instance, researchers might consider how components of the EBT might be optimally combined with psychedelic dose-administration, as previous authors have proposed.[13,64] For a ground-up approach which aims to develop a new psychological treatment component specifically for the purposes of PAT, researchers should develop clearly defined hypotheses regarding psychological mechanisms of change, how they may be augmented by psychedelic treatment, and how change processes lead to therapeutic effects in specific symptom domains. For instance, one proposed transdiagnostic drug-agnostic PAT, EMBARK, clearly outlines 6 clinical domains that therapists can target to promote benefit, which have been derived from existing empirical and qualitative evidence of psychedelic experience.[6] This model along with others of its kind[13,14] remain in need of additional empirical support that demonstrates clear relationships between intervention approaches, proposed mechanisms of change, and specific therapeutic outcomes. Like dismantling studies of combined cognitive and exposure-based interventions that have attempted to tease apart the contributions of each in promoting therapeutic change, similar approaches could be utilized in PATs to validate specific psychological intervention approaches in promoting change in theoretically relevant clinical outcome domains via well-defined mediators. This would provide confirmatory evidence for the hypothesized mechanism alone and in interaction with drug administration.

Measuring the Impact of Psychotherapy

Based on the existing evidence base, which demonstrates a striking absence of comparisons of psychological interventions in the context of drug administration, it is impossible to empirically determine the specific therapeutic contribution of the psychological component—as separate from drug and/or drug expectancy effect or in interaction with it—on symptomatic relief following PAT. Take the case of MDMA-AT for PTSD, where the placebo condition demonstrated substantial reductions in PTSD symptoms in the first Phase 3 trial.[3] Despite the intuition to deduce that this psychotherapy may be an efficacious standalone treatment, the psychological intervention needs to be tested in the absence of drug expectancy effects (which were present across all MDMA trials) to definitively establish efficacy of the psychological component utilized. Given the potential magnitude of therapeutic effects related to nonspecific relational factors (eg, rapport, therapeutic alliance) on acute outcomes in psychotherapy clinical trials, long-term measurement of symptom outcomes (eg, 6–12 months after treatment cessation) is also needed to infer whether such a standalone treatment approach is worthy of potential clinical implementation beyond EBTs already implemented in clinical practice.

Therefore, it is incumbent on clinical researchers to design trials whereby therapeutic effects can be disentangled and attributed to the drug, the psychological component, or the 2 in interaction. There are several ways in which this might be accomplished. One is to adopt a two-by-two factorial design including the following treatment arms: (1) drug and psychotherapy, (2) placebo and psychotherapy, (3) drug and no therapy, and (4) placebo and no therapy. This design would isolate the main effect of therapy (loosely defined here as any psychological component provided by trained facilitators) across drug conditions, the main effect of the drug across therapy conditions, and their interaction effect. Of the 44 reviewed studies, only one employed this full factorial design, but it was not adequately powered to assess the drug × therapy interaction effect.[33]

There are significant ethical and pragmatic challenges to this type of design, as a no-therapy condition may not be feasible for safety reasons. Therefore, researchers might instead compare an EBT such as CBT against safety-related psychological support. Given recent FDA guidance on development of psychedelics as therapeutics, it remains unlikely any psychedelic treatment would be approved without provision of some type of basic psychological support component. Consequently, the question of whether the addition of EBTs to the PAT model has any incremental additive benefit on acute and long-term clinical outcomes remains in need of empirical study. Given the high cost and implementation challenges already associated with the PAT treatment approach, it is critically important that inclusion of additional EBT components likely to raise the implementation and financial cost and provider burden associated with PAT delivery be rigorously justified based upon evidence demonstrating incremental therapeutic benefit either acutely or in the long-term. In the absence of such evidence for incremental benefit, it would be detrimental to the development and dissemination of these treatments to build in such a component for regulatory approval based upon clinical intuition alone.

SUMMARY

The present systematic review aimed to document, summarize, and constructively critique the current landscape of psychological interventions currently in use in modern psychedelic drug trials. The evidence base indicates large variability in psychological interventions used across trials, the lack of appropriate study designs to disentangle the effect of the psychological component as distinct from or in interaction with the drug or drug expectancy effect, and no clear inference on the optimal or necessary psychological treatment components to be paired with a psychedelic for any indication. We offer the following recommendations to guide research in this area. First, it will be helpful to determine the efficacy of the psychological component (if not already established) apart from any participant expectancy for or receipt of drug to eliminate the influence of drug expectancy and drug effects, respectively. These currently taint existing findings from clinical trials of psychedelic compounds with inactive placebo, active placebo, or low-dose comparator arms. Whether efficacious as a standalone treatment or not, further testing of the psychological component in interaction with an active drug can then be conducted with this important knowledge in hand. Second, experimental designs that unravel the relative contributions of PAT components are necessary to better inform treatment development, particularly in the case where researchers choose to incorporate EBTs into PAT. The optimal approach from a regulatory, treatment development, and treatment dissemination framework is to determine what is essential versus incremental versus nonincremental in optimizing therapeutic outcomes for patients, which can be most readily accomplished through rigorous validation of the incremental benefit of added components. Third, comparative efficacy and mechanism-focused trials will help to inform on how and why certain EBT components may enhance therapeutic outcomes, how such enhancements occur, and better substantiate the evidence base for novel PAT-specific psychological approaches with purported active ingredients. In aggregate, extensive foundational work needs to be undertaken to best understand how to combine psychedelics with psychotherapeutic interventions for optimal therapeutic outcomes.

CLINICS CARE POINTS

- Inform patients of the known risks and experimental status of psychedelic treatments and explore their motivations for use, treatment history, and attempt to identify other known EBTs that may be appropriate.

- If a patient appears appropriate for PAT, make patients aware that ketamine is currently the only drug approved for routine, non-research use. Consider both research trials and non-research options in treatment planning.

- If a patient elects to receive a psychedelic treatment in an approved clinical or research setting, carefully consider whether and how EBTs may be implemented to maximize the benefit.

FUNDING

GAF was supported by grants R01MH129694 and R01MH132784 from the National Institues of Health, as well as grant funding from the SEAL Future Foundation and One Mind - Baszucki Brain Research Fund.

DISCLOSURE

Dr. G A. Fonzo has received monetary compensation for consulting work with SynapseBio AI, and he owns equity in Alto Neuroscience. Neither of these activities are related to the content of this work. All of the other authors report no commercial or financial conflicts of interest.

REFERENCES

1. Nichols DE. Psychedelics. Pharmacol Rev 2016;68(2):264–355.
2. Goodwin GM, Aaronson ST, Alvarez O, et al. Single-dose psilocybin for a treatment-resistant episode of major depression. N Engl J Med 2022;387(18): 1637–48.
3. Mitchell JM, Bogenschutz M, Lilienstein A, et al. MDMA-assisted therapy for severe PTSD: a randomized, double-blind, placebo-controlled phase 3 study. Nat Med 2021;27(6):1025–33.
4. Bogenschutz MP, Ross S, Bhatt S, et al. Percentage of heavy drinking days following psilocybin-assisted psychotherapy vs placebo in the treatment of adult patients with alcohol use disorder: a randomized clinical trial. JAMA Psychiatr 2022;79(10):953–62.
5. Johnson MW, Garcia-Romeu A, Cosimano MP, et al. Pilot study of the 5-HT2AR agonist psilocybin in the treatment of tobacco addiction. J Psychopharmacol Oxf Engl 2014;28(11):983–92.
6. Brennan W, Belser AB. Models of psychedelic-assisted psychotherapy: a contemporary assessment and an introduction to embark, a transdiagnostic, trans-drug model. Front Psychol 2022;13:866018.
7. Horton DM, Morrison B, Schmidt J. Systematized Review of Psychotherapeutic Components of Psilocybin-Assisted Psychotherapy. Am J Psychother 2021; 74(4):140–9.
8. Cavarra M, Falzone A, Ramaekers JG, et al. Psychedelic-assisted psychotherapy—a systematic review of associated psychological interventions. Available at: Front Psychol 2022;13 https://www.frontiersin.org/articles/10.3389/fpsyg. 2022.887255. [Accessed 26 August 2023].
9. Mathai DS, Mora V, Garcia-Romeu A. Toward Synergies of Ketamine and Psychotherapy. Available at: Front Psychol 2022;13 https://www.frontiersin.org/articles/ 10.3389/fpsyg.2022.868103. [Accessed 28 September 2023].
10. Romeo B, Hermand M, Pétillion A, et al. Clinical and biological predictors of psychedelic response in the treatment of psychiatric and addictive disorders: A systematic review. J Psychiatr Res 2021;137:273–82.
11. Roseman L, Nutt DJ, Carhart-Harris RL. Quality of Acute Psychedelic Experience Predicts Therapeutic Efficacy of Psilocybin for Treatment-Resistant Depression. Front Pharmacol 2018;8:974.
12. Murphy R, Kettner H, Zeifman R, et al. Therapeutic Alliance and Rapport Modulate Responses to Psilocybin Assisted Therapy for Depression. Front Pharmacol 2021;12:788155.
13. Sloshower J, Guss J, Krause R, et al. Psilocybin-assisted therapy of major depressive disorder using Acceptance and Commitment Therapy as a therapeutic frame. J Context Behav Sci 2020;15:12–9.
14. Watts R, Luoma JB. The use of the psychological flexibility model to support psychedelic assisted therapy. J Context Behav Sci 2020;15:92–102.

15. Goodwin GM, Malievskaia E, Fonzo GA, et al. Must Psilocybin Always "Assist Psychotherapy". Am J Psychiatr 2023. appi.ajp.20221043. doi:10.1176/appi.ajp.20221043.
16. Fordham B, Sugavanam T, Edwards K, et al. The evidence for cognitive behavioural therapy in any condition, population or context: a meta-review of systematic reviews and panoramic meta-analysis. Psychol Med 2021;51(1):21–9.
17. Frost H, Campbell P, Maxwell M, et al. Effectiveness of Motivational Interviewing on adult behaviour change in health and social care settings: A systematic review of reviews. PLoS One 2018;13(10):e0204890.
18. Lai J, Song H, Ren Y, et al. Effectiveness of Supportive-Expressive Group Therapy in Women with Breast Cancer: A Systematic Review and Meta-Analysis. Oncol Res Treat 2021;44(5):252–60.
19. Bogenschutz MP, Forcehimes AA, Pommy JA, et al. Psilocybin-assisted treatment for alcohol dependence: a proof-of-concept study. J Psychopharmacol Oxf Engl 2015;29(3):289–99.
20. Anderson BT, Danforth A, Daroff PR, et al. Psilocybin-assisted group therapy for demoralized older long-term AIDS survivor men: An open-label safety and feasibility pilot study. EClinicalMedicine 2020;27:100538.
21. Panos PT, Jackson JW, Hasan O, et al. Meta-Analysis and Systematic Review Assessing the Efficacy of Dialectical Behavior Therapy (DBT). Res Soc Work Pract 2014;24(2):213–23.
22. Liebman RE, Whitfield KM, Sijercic I, et al. Harnessing the Healing Power of Relationships in Trauma Recovery: a Systematic Review of Cognitive-Behavioral Conjoint Therapy for PTSD. Curr Treat Options Psychiatry 2020;7(3):203–20.
23. Danforth AL, Grob CS, Struble C, et al. Reduction in social anxiety after MDMA-assisted psychotherapy with autistic adults: a randomized, double-blind, placebo-controlled pilot study. Psychopharmacology (Berl) 2018;235(11):3137–48.
24. Monson CM, Wagner AC, Mithoefer AT, et al. MDMA-facilitated cognitive-behavioural conjoint therapy for posttraumatic stress disorder: an uncontrolled trial. Eur J Psychotraumatol 2020;11(1):1840123.
25. Grant S, Colaiaco B, Motala A, et al. Mindfulness-based Relapse Prevention for Substance Use Disorders: A Systematic Review and Meta-analysis. J Addiction Med 2017;11(5):386–96.
26. McLean CP, Levy HC, Miller ML, et al. Exposure therapy for PTSD: A meta-analysis. Clin Psychol Rev 2022;91:102115.
27. Ferrando C, Selai C. A systematic review and meta-analysis on the effectiveness of exposure and response prevention therapy in the treatment of Obsessive-Compulsive Disorder. J Obsessive-Compuls Relat Disord. 2021;31:100684.
28. Rodriguez CI, Wheaton M, Zwerling J, et al. Can exposure-based CBT extend the effects of intravenous ketamine in obsessive-compulsive disorder? an open-label trial. J Clin Psychiatry 2016;77(3):408–9.
29. Shiroma P, McManus E, Voller E, et al. Repeated Sub-Anesthetic Ketamine to Enhance Prolonged Exposure Therapy in Post-Traumatic Stress Disorder: A Proof-Of-Concept Study. Biol Psychiatry 2020;87(9):S217.
30. Wilkinson ST, Wright D, Fasula MK, et al. Cognitive Behavior Therapy May Sustain Antidepressant Effects of Intravenous Ketamine in Treatment-Resistant Depression. Psychother Psychosom 2017;86(3):162–7.
31. Wilkinson ST, Rhee TG, Joormann J, et al. Cognitive Behavioral Therapy to Sustain the Antidepressant Effects of Ketamine in Treatment-Resistant Depression: A Randomized Clinical Trial. Psychother Psychosom 2021;90(5):318–27.

32. Dakwar E, Levin F, Hart CL, et al. A Single Ketamine Infusion Combined With Motivational Enhancement Therapy for Alcohol Use Disorder: A Randomized Midazolam-Controlled Pilot Trial. Am J Psychiatr 2020;177(2):125–33.
33. Grabski M, McAndrew A, Lawn W, et al. Adjunctive Ketamine With Relapse Prevention-Based Psychological Therapy in the Treatment of Alcohol Use Disorder. Am J Psychiatr 2022;179(2):152–62.
34. Dakwar E, Nunes EV, Hart CL, et al. A Single Ketamine Infusion Combined With Mindfulness-Based Behavioral Modification to Treat Cocaine Dependence: A Randomized Clinical Trial. Am J Psychiatr 2019;176(11):923–30.
35. Azhari N, Hu H, O'Malley KY, et al. Ketamine-facilitated behavioral treatment for cannabis use disorder: A proof of concept study. Am J Drug Alcohol Abuse 2021;47(1):92–7.
36. Ross S, Bossis A, Guss J, et al. Rapid and sustained symptom reduction following psilocybin treatment for anxiety and depression in patients with life-threatening cancer: a randomized controlled trial. J Psychopharmacol Oxf Engl 2016;30(12):1165–80.
37. Carhart-Harris R, Giribaldi B, Watts R, et al. Trial of Psilocybin versus Escitalopram for Depression. N Engl J Med 2021;384(15):1402–11.
38. Goodwin GM, Croal M, Feifel D, et al. Psilocybin for treatment resistant depression in patients taking a concomitant SSRI medication. Neuropsychopharmacology 2023;48(10):1492–9.
39. Schneier FR, Feusner J, Wheaton MG, et al. Pilot study of single-dose psilocybin for serotonin reuptake inhibitor-resistant body dysmorphic disorder. J Psychiatr Res 2023;161:364–70.
40. Sloshower J, Skosnik PD, Safi-Aghdam H, et al. Psilocybin-assisted therapy for major depressive disorder: An exploratory placebo-controlled, fixed-order trial. J Psychopharmacol Oxf Engl 2023;37(7):698–706.
41. Moreno FA, Wiegand CB, Taitano EK, et al. Safety, tolerability, and efficacy of psilocybin in 9 patients with obsessive-compulsive disorder. J Clin Psychiatry 2006;67(11):1735–40.
42. Grob CS, Danforth AL, Chopra GS, et al. Pilot study of psilocybin treatment for anxiety in patients with advanced-stage cancer. Arch Gen Psychiatry 2011;68(1):71–8.
43. Griffiths RR, Johnson MW, Carducci MA, et al. Psilocybin produces substantial and sustained decreases in depression and anxiety in patients with life-threatening cancer: A randomized double-blind trial. J Psychopharmacol Oxf Engl 2016;30(12):1181–97.
44. Carhart-Harris RL, Bolstridge M, Rucker J, et al. Psilocybin with psychological support for treatment-resistant depression: an open-label feasibility study. Lancet Psychiatr 2016;3(7):619–27.
45. Davis AK, Barrett FS, May DG, et al. Effects of Psilocybin-Assisted Therapy on Major Depressive Disorder: A Randomized Clinical Trial. JAMA Psychiatr 2021;78(5):481–9.
46. Shnayder S, Ameli R, Sinaii N, et al. Psilocybin-assisted therapy improves psychosocial-spiritual well-being in cancer patients. J Affect Disord 2023;323:592–7.
47. von Rotz R, Schindowski EM, Jungwirth J, et al. Single-dose psilocybin-assisted therapy in major depressive disorder: A placebo-controlled, double-blind, randomised clinical trial. eClinicalMedicine 2023;56. von Rotz R., robin.vonrotz@bli.uzh.ch; Schindowski E.M.; Jungwirth J.; Schuldt A.; Rieser N.M.; Zahoranszky K.; Preller K.H.; Vollenweider F.X.) Neurophenomenology of

Consciousness Lab, Department of Psychiatry, Psychotherapy and Psychosomatics, Psychiatric Hospital, University of Zurich, Zürich, Switzerland).

48. Mithoefer MC, Mithoefer AT, Feduccia AA, et al. 3,4-methylenedioxymethamphetamine (MDMA)-assisted psychotherapy for post-traumatic stress disorder in military veterans, firefighters, and police officers: a randomised, double-blind, dose-response, phase 2 clinical trial. Lancet Psychiatr 2018;5(6):486–97.

49. Mithoefer MC, Wagner MT, Mithoefer AT, et al. The safety and efficacy of {+/-}3,4-methylenedioxymethamphetamine-assisted psychotherapy in subjects with chronic, treatment-resistant posttraumatic stress disorder: the first randomized controlled pilot study. J Psychopharmacol Oxf Engl 2011;25(4):439–52.

50. Jardim AV, Jardim DV, Chaves BR, et al. 3,4-methylenedioxymethamphetamine (MDMA)-assisted psychotherapy for victims of sexual abuse with severe posttraumatic stress disorder: an open label pilot study in Brazil. Braz J Psychiatry 2021;43(2):181–5.

51. Ot'alora GM, Grigsby J, Poulter B, et al. 3,4-Methylenedioxymethamphetamine-assisted psychotherapy for treatment of chronic posttraumatic stress disorder: A randomized phase 2 controlled trial. J Psychopharmacol Oxf Engl 2018;32(12):1295–307.

52. Oehen P, Traber R, Widmer V, et al. A randomized, controlled pilot study of MDMA (± 3,4-Methylenedioxymethamphetamine)-assisted psychotherapy for treatment of resistant, chronic Post-Traumatic Stress Disorder (PTSD). J Psychopharmacol Oxf Engl 2013;27(1):40–52.

53. Bouso JC, Doblin R, Farré M, et al. MDMA-assisted psychotherapy using low doses in a small sample of women with chronic posttraumatic stress disorder. J Psychoact Drugs 2008;40(3):225–36.

54. Wolfson PE, Andries J, Feduccia AA, et al. MDMA-assisted psychotherapy for treatment of anxiety and other psychological distress related to life-threatening illnesses: a randomized pilot study. Sci Rep 2020;10(1):20442.

55. Sessa B, Higbed L, O'Brien S, et al. First study of safety and tolerability of 3,4-methylenedioxymethamphetamine-assisted psychotherapy in patients with alcohol use disorder. J Psychopharmacol Oxf Engl 2021;35(4):375–83.

56. Krupitsky EM, Burakov AM, Dunaevsky IV, et al. Single versus repeated sessions of ketamine-assisted psychotherapy for people with heroin dependence. J Psychoact Drugs 2007;39(1):13–9.

57. Pradhan B, Mitrev L, Moaddell R, et al. D-Serine is a potential biomarker for clinical response in treatment of post-traumatic stress disorder using (R,S)-ketamine infusion and TIMBER psychotherapy: A pilot study. Biochim Biophys Acta, Proteins Proteomics 2018;1866(7):831–9.

58. Price RB, Spotts C, Panny B, et al. A Novel, Brief, Fully Automated Intervention to Extend the Antidepressant Effect of a Single Ketamine Infusion: A Randomized Clinical Trial. Am J Psychiatr 2022;179(12):959–68.

59. Palhano-Fontes F, Barreto D, Onias H, et al. Rapid antidepressant effects of the psychedelic ayahuasca in treatment-resistant depression: a randomized placebo-controlled trial. Psychol Med 2019;49(4):655–63.

60. Dos Santos RG, Rocha JM, Rossi GN, et al. Effects of ayahuasca on the endocannabinoid system of healthy volunteers and in volunteers with social anxiety disorder: Results from two pilot, proof-of-concept, randomized, placebo-controlled trials. Hum Psychopharmacol 2022;37(4):e2834.

61. Gasser P, Holstein D, Michel Y, et al. Safety and efficacy of lysergic acid diethylamide-assisted psychotherapy for anxiety associated with life-threatening diseases. J Nerv Ment Dis 2014;202(7):513–20.

62. Holze F, Gasser P, Müller F, et al. Lysergic Acid Diethylamide-Assisted Therapy in Patients With Anxiety With and Without a Life-Threatening Illness: A Randomized, Double-Blind, Placebo-Controlled Phase II Study. Biol Psychiatry 2023;93(3): 215–23.

63. D'Souza D, Syed SA, Flynn LT, et al. Multisite Randomized, Double-Blind, Placebo-Controlled, Parallel Group Study of the Efficacy, Safety and Tolerability of the Fatty Acid Amide Hydrolase (FAAH) Inhibitor JZP150 (PF-04457845) in Adults With Cannabis Use Disorder (CUD). Neuropsychopharmacology 2022;47. D'Souza D.) Yale University, School of Medicine, West Haven, CT, United States):35.

64. Yaden DB, Earp D, Graziosi M, et al. Psychedelics and Psychotherapy: Cognitive-Behavioral Approaches as Default. Available at: Front Psychol 2022; 13 https://www.frontiersin.org/articles/10.3389/fpsyg.2022.873279. [Accessed 25 September 2023].

Technology-based Cognitive Behavioral Therapy Interventions

Jill M. Newby, PhD[a,b,c],*, Emily Upton, M. Psych (Clinical)[c],
Elizabeth Mason, PhD[d], Melissa Black, PhD[b,c]

KEYWORDS

- Internet-delivered cognitive behavioral therapy • E-Health interventions • Anxiety
- Mood disorders • Smartphone apps • Digital cognitive behavioral therapy

KEY POINTS

- Technology can increase access to cognitive behavioral therapy (CBT), overcoming barriers to care.
- Examples include guided and unguided Internet and app-based CBT, and telehealth CBT.
- Internet CBT is effective in treating depression and anxiety disorders.
- Emerging evidence for smartphone app-based CBT for depression and anxiety.

INTRODUCTION/BACKGROUND

Technology has become increasingly important in mental health care, enabling individuals and their loved ones to easily access free or low-cost mental health information, self-help tools and advice, support groups, screening, and evidence-based treatments such as cognitive behavioral therapy (CBT). Despite decades of evidence supporting the use of CBT in the treatment of a range of mental health conditions, CBT is not always readily accessible or affordable to access. A range of barriers to accessing CBT exist, including high cost of treatment, stigma, lack of knowledge and awareness of CBT, and shortage of skilled CBT practitioners. Individual factors such as caring responsibilities and mobility issues can make it difficult to attend in-person CBT clinics, and geographic restrictions can require long, expensive, and impractical distances to travel. These barriers disproportionately affect people living

[a] UNSW at the Black Dog Institute, Hospital Road, Randwick, New South Wales 2031, Australia;
[b] School of Psychology, UNSW Sydney; [c] Black Dog Institute, Hospital Road, Randwick, New
South Wales 2031, Australia; [d] Clinical Research Unit for Anxiety and Depression, St Vincent's
Health Network, Level 4 O'Brien Centre, St Vincent's Hospital, Victoria Street, Corner Burton
Street, Darlinghurst, New South Wales 2010, Australia
* Corresponding author. UNSW at the Black Dog Institute, Hospital Road, Randwick, New
South Wales 2031, Australia.
E-mail address: j.newby@unsw.edu.au

Psychiatr Clin N Am 47 (2024) 399–417
https://doi.org/10.1016/j.psc.2024.02.004
0193-953X/24/© 2024 Elsevier Inc. All rights reserved.

in rural, regional, and remote areas, carers, and people from lower socioeconomic backgrounds.

Over the past 20 years, innovations in technology, such as the use of web sites, smartphone apps, and tablets, telephones, and video-conferencing have been used to deliver CBT. Technology can help improve equitable access to affordable and high-quality mental health care, overcoming barriers to treatment. Without the need to travel to appointments, individuals can access convenient treatment, which is often more affordable than face-to-face care, and can be accessed outside of traditional office hours (eg, 9 am–5 pm). Technology helps ensure treatment is standardized and consistent across patients, and in-built patient-reported outcome monitoring can help track patient progress, allowing early response to symptom deterioration. In countries and settings where the mental health workforce is limited, especially in rural, regional, and remote areas, technology can help fill the workforce shortage of CBT practitioners.

AIMS OF THE STUDY

This review focuses on the use of technology-based CBT interventions in adults. The aims of this study are 3 fold. First, we describe the main types of technology-based CBT interventions. Second, we describe the latest evidence from randomized controlled trials (RCTs), systematic reviews, and meta-analyses of technology-based CBT for the treatment of a range of mental health conditions. Third, we describe gaps in the research and potential future directions in the field.

WHAT DO TECHNOLOGY-BASED COGNITIVE BEHAVIORAL THERAPY INTERVENTIONS INVOLVE?

A wide range of technology-delivered CBT interventions have been developed. In this review, we focus on CBT delivered via the Internet, smartphone apps, and telehealth (phone or videoconferencing).

These technology-based CBT programs typically provide the core foundations of CBT education and skills, including

- Psychoeducation about the presenting problem;
- Self-monitoring (eg, mood monitoring, self-report questionnaires to track symptom change);
- Goal setting;
- Cognitive therapy techniques such as thought monitoring, thought challenging, and behavioral experiments;
- Behavioral therapy techniques such as behavioral activation, problem solving, and graded exposure;
- Other techniques such as relaxation, mindfulness and acceptance techniques; and
- Relapse prevention.

Technology-delivered CBT interventions can vary widely in the way they are implemented and used. While the core CBT components are delivered through technology, they may differ in the platform on which they are available (such as mobile smartphone application, tablets, open or closed websites available on personal computers), the countries and languages they are available, program duration, their costs, and the nature and type of guidance provided. Programs can range from completely unguided/ self-guided online interventions, to blended care models which combine digital and in-person therapy, to synchronous CBT sessions delivered in real time, by a trained mental health professional. We define common examples as follows:

- Unguided or guided Internet-delivered CBT (iCBT; see Refs[1,2]):
  - In *an unguided or self-guided internet CBT program,* an individual will work through the program on their own without the support of a coach or therapist. They might read through online modules and complete CBT homework tasks alone, either without feedback or with fully automated feedback from the program. Some unguided programs include technical support from a human, but most are done completely without support.
  - In guided Internet CBT programs, trained coaches or mental health professionals (eg, psychologists, trainee psychologists, psychiatrists) provide remote support to the individual as they work through the online program. Guided Internet CBT programs vary in the amount, nature, and extent of therapist support, and whether the support is in real time (synchronous) or asynchronous. Some include regular phone calls, while others provide written feedback on homework tasks, and some involve automated SMS reminders. Some may include email support and check-ins, phone calls, video chat, SMSs, or written feedback through web-portals which are asynchronous. This support can range from technical support and troubleshooting to motivation and engagement support, to more sophisticated therapeutic work and advice from a therapist. Some are scheduled at specific times and others are on demand (as needed).
- Blended CBT treatment[3] involves the digital component supporting in-person individual or group-based CBT sessions. Digital components could be online modules or progress tracking between sessions, either as an add-on to traditional therapy or to replace certain parts of the same treatment protocol.
- Smartphone app-based CBT can either be guided or unguided, as with Internet CBT programs. However, the CBT components are delivered via smartphone apps, rather than on a web site. Some recent apps have been developed with Chatbot that aim to provide support, encouragement, and feedback, though most research has been done on human-supported or unguided app-based CBT.
- CBT delivered via telehealth. In this study, telehealth refers to the delivery of synchronous treatment via telephone or videoconference. Synchronous telehealth allows real-time interaction between patient and provider and is more similar to in-person treatment compared to asynchronous support from a health care provider.

INTERNET-DELIVERED COGNITIVE BEHAVIORAL THERAPY

The most widely researched technology-based CBT intervention is internet-assisted or internet-delivered CBT (see Ref[2]). Next we summarize recent evidence from reviews of published randomized trials and meta-analyses of Internet CBT for the treatment of common mental health conditions in adults.

EFFECTS ON DEPRESSION

A large number of RCTs and meta-analyses have been conducted on Internet-delivered CBT for depression, including people with elevated depressive symptoms and diagnosed depressive disorders.[4] Overall, these studies show moderate-to-large effect sizes compared to control groups,[5] with good acceptability by patients including satisfaction and adherence.[5] The methodological quality of studies is generally reported to be good with low risk of bias.[5,6] In one meta-analysis, Andrews and colleagues[5] found moderate differences compared to controls from 32 RCTs comparing Internet CBT to wait list or usual care control groups (effect size = 0.67). Studies also show good evidence for transdiagnostic Internet CBT for mixed depressive and anxiety disorders (eg, see Ref[7]).

Comparisons of therapist-guided Internet CBT and face-to-face CBT have shown little difference in effect size (n = 5, effect size = −0.21 [-0.58–0.16][8]), or patient satisfaction but iCBT costs less to deliver.[9] A systematic review and Individual Patient Data Network Meta-analysis found that both guided and unguided Internet CBTs were more effective in treating depression than control treatments over the short and long term, with treatment gains maintained at 6 and 12 month follow up across many studies.[6] Individual patient meta-analyses have revealed that for mild or subthreshold depression, both guided and unguided Internet CBT programs are effective. For moderate-to-severe depression, however, guided Internet CBT is more effective than unguided Internet CBT. Overall, these results show strong evidence for the efficacy of Internet CBT in depression treatment, and indicate the use of guided programs for moderate-to-severe depression.

EFFECTS ON ANXIETY AND RELATED DISORDERS

The largest body of research into technology-based CBT interventions is focused on anxiety and related disorders. In a pooled analysis of RCTs comparing Internet CBT for anxiety disorders to inactive controls, Pauley and colleagues[10] found large differences of 0.8 favoring digital CBT over controls, with good evidence of data quality and validity. Of 9 comparisons between digital and face-to-face CBTs, there was no difference in outcomes. These treatments also have evidence of good acceptability and adherence rates in patients.[5]

Research shows that Internet CBT is more effective than control groups in the treatment of generalized anxiety disorder (GAD),[11] panic disorder and agoraphobia,[12] social anxiety disorder (SAD),[5] severe health anxiety,[13] and obsessive compulsive disorder (OCD).[14] Evidence is emerging for Internet CBT for post-traumatic stress disorder (PTSD), with small-to-moderate differences relative to control groups. Several transdiagnostic Internet CBT interventions for multiple anxiety disorders (and anxiety disorders with comorbid depression) have also been shown to be effective, with small effect sizes in favor of transdiagnostic over disorder-specific Internet CBT interventions.[15–17]

EFFECTS ON GENERALIZED ANXIETY DISORDER

In a meta-analysis of 9 RCTs, Andrews and colleagues[5] found a moderate difference (0.70) between disorder-specific Internet CBT programs for GAD compared to inactive controls. A more recent meta-analysis by Eilert and colleagues[11] included both disorder-specific and transdiagnostic Internet CBT for GAD. They[11] found moderate-to-large effect sizes compared to controls for anxiety (0.79) and worry (0.75) as well as depression (0.70), and a small-to-moderate effect size for quality of life and functional impairment (0.33), with likely maintenance of gains at follow up and high rates of program completion. Studies were generally of good methodological quality.[11]

EFFECTS ON SOCIAL ANXIETY DISORDER (SOCIAL PHOBIA)

In one meta-analysis of 11 RCTs of internet CBT for social anxiety disorder (formerly social phobia), a large difference was found compared to controls (0.92[5]). A recent systematic review and meta-analysis of 20 trials found that Internet CBT significantly reduced symptoms of SAD, outperforming control groups with moderate differences in social anxiety (0.55), and gains maintained at 6 and 12 month follow up.[18] It also produces equivalent effects to in-person CBT (0.18) but may be more acceptable than face-to-face CBT for patients as the therapist themselves may be a phobic object.[18]

EFFECTS ON PANIC DISORDER AND/OR AGORAPHOBIA

In a meta-analysis of 12 RCTs, large effect sizes were found comparing Internet CBT to control groups (effect size of 1.31).[5] Another meta-analysis of the effects of Internet CBT for panic disorder and/or agoraphobia[12] found large differences between Internet CBT and controls from 9 RCTs on panic symptoms (1.22) and agoraphobia (0.91), which were maintained at 3 and 6 month follow-up. Methodological quality of trials and adherence rates varied across studies, but advantages of iCBT over control remained significant even after lower-quality studies were removed from the meta-analysis; nevertheless, further high-quality studies on iCBT for panic and agoraphobia are needed.[12]

EFFECTS ON OBSESSIVE COMPULSIVE DISORDER

Less research has been done in Internet CBT-based treatment of OCD compared to other anxiety disorders. In a review and meta-analysis of 6 RCTs, Machado-Sousa et al.[14] found large overall effect sizes for Internet CBT for OCD treatments compared to controls (0.81), with treatment gains maintained at follow-up. Adherence varied across studies but therapist guidance helped reduce drop-out.[14] While further high-quality trials are needed, it appears that delivering CBT for OCD online significantly improves access to specialist treatment that is often difficult to access for this population.[14,19]

EFFECTS ON SEVERE HEALTH ANXIETY

There are no systematic reviews and meta-analyses of Internet CBT for health anxiety specifically. However, guided Internet CBT has been shown to significantly improve severe health anxiety with large differences compared to a range of control groups including wait list, anxiety psychoeducation, and stress management, with gains maintained at follow-up,[20–22] and benefits compared to control such as higher treatment satisfaction[20] and adherence.[21] One recent RCT found Internet CBT was noninferior to individual face-to-face CBT for health anxiety but with significantly lower costs.[23]

EFFECTS ON POST-TRAUMATIC STRESS DISORDER

There are initial promising results for Interned-based CBT for PTSD in military/veteran, public safety personnel, and general populations, but due to the small number of studies conducted, further research is needed with bigger samples and to compare the results with face-to-face CBT. One review identified 10 trials and found moderate differences in reduction of PTSD symptoms compared to wait list controls (standardized mean difference [SMD] = 0.60).[24] However, they also reported that the quality of evidence was low, and there is little data on longer term outcomes with no evidence so far to show maintenance of improvement at follow-up of 3 to 6 months. Another review focused solely on PTSD treatment in veterans,[25] and found 6 RCTs, with small effects in favor of Internet CBT for PTSD over controls (SMD = 0.29), although some trials included had very small samples so further research is needed.

EFFECTS OF INTERNET CBT FOR DEPRESSION AND ANXIETY IN SPECIFIC POPULATIONS

Most research testing Internet CBT for depression and anxiety has been designed for adults in the general population. However, several RCTs show that Internet CBT is also beneficial for symptoms of depression and anxiety in the perinatal period,[26] including in pregnancy[27] and the postpartum period.[28,29] Research trials also show that Internet CBT improves depression and anxiety in people with comorbid chronic conditions including Type 1 and 2 diabetes,[30] early stage cancer,[31] and osteoarthritis.[32] In one review, Mehta and colleagues[33] explored the efficacy of Internet CBT for depression and anxiety in patients with conditions such as chronic pain, tinnitus, and rheumatoid arthritis. They found significant improvements in symptoms as a result of Internet CBT, and larger effect sizes were seen for guided versus unguided Internet CBT.

EFFECTS ON INSOMNIA

Internet CBT for insomnia is a multicomponent treatment which includes psychoeducation, sleep hygiene, stimulus control, sleep restriction, cognitive therapy, and relaxation training (see Ref[34]). There is strong evidence for the effectiveness of digital CBT in treating insomnia with research studies of generally good quality.[35] A recent meta-analysis of 11 RCTs found a large post-treatment effect size for insomnia severity ($g = 1.09$), a medium effect size for sleep efficiency (the time spent in bed asleep; $g = 0.59$), and a small effect on sleep quality, time taken to fall asleep, and the number and duration of night time awakenings (g's = 0.21–0.49).[35] A meta-analysis of 33 RCTs (11 included follow-up assessments) found that improvements in insomnia symptoms are maintained up to 1 year follow-up.[36] Direct comparisons have shown that digital CBT for insomnia achieves similar treatment effects to therapist-delivered CBT, but may be more cost-effective due to the lower costs of delivery.[37–39] Adherence rates in iCBT for insomnia tend to vary across studies,[35] but this also applies to research on face-to-face CBT for insomnia[40]; more research is needed to ascertain factors determining adherence. Digital CBT for insomnia has also been shown to be effective for specific groups, including pregnant women. For example, Kalmbach and colleagues[41] showed it improves sleep quality and sleep duration during pregnancy and after childbirth. Studies show interesting positive effects of digital CBT beyond insomnia to comorbid symptoms. For example, digital CBT for insomnia has also been shown to improve anxiety and depression symptoms[42,43] and prevent depression.[44]

EFFECTS ON EATING DISORDERS

The evidence for the acceptability and efficacy of technology-based interventions for eating disorders is limited, with far fewer trials than other mental health conditions and inconsistent results across studies. Despite some promising preliminary results for some symptoms (eg, reduction of binge eating in binge eating disorder and bulimia nervosa), many studies show poor acceptability and adherence rates to guided and self-help Internet CBT in eating disorder samples. In one review of Internet CBT for full or subthreshold binge eating disorder, Moghimi and colleagues[45] identified only 3 trials. Their preliminary findings suggested small-to-moderate differences compared with waitlist controls in improving binge eating episodes, and eating disorder symptomology, but no differences in changes in body mass index between Internet CBT and controls. In another systematic review focused on all eating disorders, Ahmadiankalati and colleagues[46] identified 12 published RCTs from 2016 to 2020. They concluded there was insufficient evidence to determine acceptability or effectiveness of these interventions compared to controls. RCTs of Internet or technology-based interventions for anorexia nervosa are lacking, likely due to the importance of medical supervision required in treatment which is difficult to conduct remotely. Direct comparisons between guided Internet CBT and face-to-face CBT for eating disorders have mostly found better outcomes in face-to-face CBT than Internet CBT, including for binge eating disorder (individual CBT[47]) and bulimia nervosa (group CBT[48]).

EFFECTS ON SUBSTANCE USE DISORDERS

Most studies of digital interventions for substance use disorders do not involve CBT,[49] and there have been no meta-analyses of Internet or technology-based CBT for substance use disorders to our knowledge.

One review of interventions for problematic cannabis use identified 5 trials of motivational interviewing combined with CBT for cannabis dependence and found small effect sizes on cannabis use.[50] In another review of Internet interventions for people with dependence on opioids, cocaine, and amphetamines, Internet CBT was found to produce small effects on the use of these substances ($n = 4$, $g = 0.19$).[51] One systematic review of Internet CBT for alcohol misuse[52] found 14 RCTs, only 2 of which required participants to fulfill the full diagnostic criteria for alcohol-use disorder (the rest only included those who screened positive for elevated alcohol use). They reported medium-to-large effects favoring therapist-guided Internet CBT compared to wait list controls for reducing alcohol use and small-to-moderate differences between therapist-guided and self-guided Internet CBT (favoring guided programs). Another review identified only 3 RCTs of digital CBT for alcohol use disorder during the period of 2016 to 2019.[53] Computer-based CBT in combination with usual care produced greater numbers of days abstinent from alcohol than usual care at post-treatment ($d = 0.71$). Overall, very few trials have been conducted, and attrition rates in Internet CBT for alcohol use range from 30% to 50%. Further research is needed to evaluate the efficacy of Internet CBT for alcohol and substance dependence.

TELEHEALTH-BASED COGNITIVE BEHAVIORAL THERAPY

Initially research into tele-based CBT focused on delivering CBT via the telephone, remotely. More recently, improvements in technologies such as Zoom, Skype, Facetime, and other types of videoconferencing software have enabled CBT sessions to be delivered remotely with the ability for the therapist and client to see each other in real time. While the initial uptake of telehealth-based CBT was slow, the COVID-19 pandemic influenced rapid adoption of this technology in practice. Several RCTs and systematic reviews have examined CBT delivered via telehealth for depression, anxiety, PTSD, and mixed diagnoses. Overall, individual and group CBT delivered via telehealth are as effective as CBT delivered in-person.[54–56] In one systematic review of 22 RCTs, comparing the effectiveness of telehealth CBT compared to in-person CBT, Bellanti and colleagues[54] found that clinical outcomes did not differ between delivery methods. Most studies also found no significant differences in satisfaction with care, therapeutic alliance, or study discontinuation between delivery methods. For depression specifically, telephone-delivered CBT was noninferior to face-to-face CBT in reducing depression symptoms, but associated with lower drop out,[57] and in another study was more cost-effective than face-to-face CBT.[58] A recent systematic review found that some telehealth groups are feasible and as effective as in-person treatment and with high participant satisfaction,[59] but few of these studies have evaluated telehealth CBT group programs for depression and/or anxiety disorders.

RESPONSE TO THE COVID-19 PANDEMIC

Technology-based CBT interventions can be rapidly deployed during pandemics, and other national emergencies. Through the COVID-19 pandemic, we saw the importance of being able to access timely, affordable, evidence-based mental health care, without the need to travel to see practitioners in person. Technology-based CBT played a significant role in the COVID-19 response, when lockdowns and other restrictions on movement made it difficult to access in-person care for nonemergency situations. It also led to rapid increases in the uptake of telehealth CBT and other interventions for mental health. One systematic review and meta-analysis found that Internet CBT significantly decreased symptoms of depression and anxiety in people during the COVID-19 pandemic.[60] Individual effectiveness studies also found considerable increase in demand for Internet CBT courses, and significant improvements in depression and anxiety that were similar in size to pre-pandemic effects.[61–63] One study found that technology-based CBT delivered via iPad was more effective than treatment as usual for treating depressive and anxiety symptoms and insomnia in people with COVID-19 (who were more at risk for these disorders but could not access face-to-face treatment while unwell).[64]

TECHNOLOGY-BASED CBT INTERVENTIONS EFFECTS GENERALIZE TO ROUTINE MENTAL HEALTH CARE SETTINGS

One of the criticisms of technology-based CBT trials has been that trials have been conducted on motivated self-referred patients who are "different" or less severe in clinical presentation compared to those seen in routine care mental health settings. Studies have shown that technology-based CBT interventions are acceptable and remain effective treatments for anxiety and depression in routine care settings, and are generalizable beyond clinical trials to multiple health care settings,[65] including in real-world teaching clinic settings.[66] However, some studies show a drop in engagement and adherence in technology-based CBT in routine care settings compared to research trials (eg, see Refs[67,68]).

WHAT FACTORS ARE ASSOCIATED WITH POSITIVE OUTCOMES IN TECHNOLOGY-BASED CBT INTERVENTIONS?
Patient Characteristics

Several reviews have summarized the literature on moderators and predictors of treatment response in technology-based CBT interventions, especially Internet CBT programs. Overall, there are few replicated findings across studies. In a recent review, Haller and colleagues[69] reported that better adherence/engagement, baseline self-report ratings of treatment credibility and expectations of benefit, and working alliance were the most reliable predictors of better outcomes. Some studies also show higher baseline severity scores on self-report measures predict larger changes in symptoms, but also higher post-treatment scores. Individual patient network analysis studies have identified that patients with more severe symptoms or greater deficits at baseline may benefit the most from Internet CBT treatment of various anxiety and depressive disorders[66]; another found that older adults and those with greater initial depression symptoms benefited the most from Internet CBT depression treatment compared to those with subthreshold depression.[70]

Therapeutic Alliance and Guidance

Several dismantling studies using individual patient-level and component-level network analysis have begun to identify the most effective elements of Internet CBT treatments, and to help match treatments to patients.[6,71] Despite some of the benefits of technology-based delivery of treatments including increased automation, neutrality, and anonymity, much of the research has found that therapist guidance and therapeutic alliance remain key elements of effective technology-based treatment. Some reviews comparing guided versus nonguided Internet CBT treatments have found superior treatment outcomes for treatments with some form of therapist guidance (eg, Refs[6,72]). Many studies have also found a positive correlation between therapeutic alliance and treatment outcome (eg, Ref[73]). High patient dropout is a key limitation of unguided technology-based CBT.[74] Therapist guidance tends to increase patient adherence and treatment completion, and reduces patient dropout.[72] Even combining human and automated encouragement tends to reduce drop out.[71] Unguided Internet CBT, however, has still been shown to be effective in several studies, and may be better suited to mild or subthreshold symptoms, or for preventative purposes.[6]

Persuasive Design

Several studies have examined ways to increase engagement in unguided Internet CBT treatments. Use of persuasive design principles (designed to facilitate task completion, and provide dialogue and social support, such as tailoring, personalization, praise, reminders, and social learning) can increase patient engagement, although there is variability in how much is used among different available treatments (see Ref[75] for full list of recommended design principles for eHealth interventions). Although the use of gamification in mental health apps is mostly intended to increase user engagement and enhance intervention effects,[76] a systematic review and meta-analysis by Six and colleagues[77] found no significant difference in the effectiveness of mental health apps with or without gamification elements on either depressive symptoms or adherence. Further research is needed to determine the most effective persuasive design elements that impact on engagement and patient outcomes.

Personalizing Treatment

A further way that may be important to increase the effectiveness of online treatments is to personalize treatment, selecting treatment type/components by individual patient. Furuwaka and colleagues[71] have developed a collaborative treatment selection tool individualized to patients' symptoms, needs, and preferences, designed to be used as a discussion tool between the patient and therapist in selecting the best-matched digital treatment. Other examples of tools that screen for symptom severity and recommend disorder-specific or transdiagnostic Internet CBT programs are also in clinical use, but have not been evaluated (eg, https://thiswayup.org.au/take-a-test-tool/).

NEGATIVE EFFECTS OF TECHNOLOGY-BASED CBT INTERVENTIONS

A relatively new and emerging field of research is exploring adverse or unwanted negative effects of Internet therapies.[78] Though studies vary, one individual patient meta-analysis of 29 trials found 5.8% will experience clinically reliable deterioration.[79] Other studies have found estimates of between 10% and 15% of patients experience some temporary negative experiences including increased distress or anxiety as a result of techniques included, including self-monitoring and exposure therapy.[80]

APP-BASED CBT INTERVENTIONS

Since the development of smartphones, the number and range of mental health and well-being apps has grown exponentially. Yet, the evidence of the efficacy of apps for the treatment of mental health conditions is still emerging. The number of studies investigating the efficacy of app-based CBT is still limited, particularly in comparison to the wealth of evidence for the efficacy of online/web-based programs,[81] and lagging far behind the availability of mental health apps. Many mental health apps with research evidence have not been made publicly available, and many apps that are publicly or commercially available lack evidence of their safety and efficacy. Several reviews of mental health apps available in app stores have found only a small fraction of publicly available mental health apps have published peer-reviewed evidence on either feasibility or efficacy (eg, 2.08%[82]). Much of the research is in the pilot or feasibility stages, so further rigorous investigation is needed.[83]

There is a lack of evidence for the use of mobile-only interventions for eating disorders[84] and PTSD[85] suggesting they should not be used as stand-alone interventions. However, mobile health apps for anxiety and depression have been found to result in small-to-medium improvements in symptoms compared to control groups.[83,86–88] Despite this promising evidence, there are challenges with the use of mobile mental health apps for treating depression and anxiety. Most RCTs have compared apps to inactive controls, which make it difficult to establish whether mental health apps outperform a "digital placebo effect."[89] Studies of app-based CBT also suffer from high rates of drop-out and disengagement.[90] Apps may be better suited to use in conjunction with or as an adjunct to other forms of therapy, to facilitate engagement with therapeutic activities, such as homework tasks between sessions.[87] Further research is needed to test the use of mobile CBT apps in blended care models, and to test the efficacy of mobile CBT interventions for other mental health conditions.

EMERGING AREAS OF RESEARCH INTO MOBILE MENTAL HEALTH APPS

There is some promising initial evidence that mobile apps for suicide prevention can have positive effects for individuals at elevated risk of suicide or self-harm, in reducing depression, psychological distress, and self-harm, and increasing coping self-efficacy, although none evaluated demonstrated the ability to significantly decrease suicidal ideation compared with a control condition.[91] RCTs are needed to determine efficacy, relative to control groups, and in-person therapy.

There are some newly developed CBT-based "Chatbots" designed to deliver CBT treatment via a substitute for human interaction showing some initial promise in terms of user engagement (eg, Ref[92]). One evaluation of an app-based CBT Chatbot treatment of panic disorder, for example, showed significant decreases in disorder severity compared to a control group.[93] However, the evidence for app-based CBT Chatbots is only emerging, in studies with small samples, and inconclusive regarding efficacy.

LIMITATIONS OF EXISTING EVIDENCE

The research literature on technology-based CBT interventions has been rapidly growing over the last few decades. Despite this, gaps in the evidence remain.

- Most clinical trials typically exclude individuals with very severe symptoms (eg, severe depression), people who are acutely suicidal, and people with psychotic disorders. Research is needed to explore the acceptability and efficacy of technology-based CBT interventions in these populations.

- Most research has been done in high-income western countries, with fewer studies conducted in low or middle income countries, or in populations from diverse cultural and ethnic backgrounds.[94] More research is needed to evaluate the acceptability, feasibility, and efficacy of culturally adapted technology-based CBT interventions in low and middle income countries.[95]
- Although emerging findings suggest little difference in efficacy between Internet and face-to-face CBT,[8] technology and face-to-face CBT have not been compared for the treatment of some mental health disorders, or have only one trial (and no replicated RCTs) to compare their effects.[8]
- Most technology-based CBT interventions require minimum reading level and educational level to understand and are not accessible or suitable to all clients (see Ref[96] for an example of an e-health program for people with intellectual disability).
- While evidence shows significant, often large improvements in symptoms, the impact of technology-supported CBT interventions on quality of life appears to be more modest (small-to-moderate effects) than the impact on symptoms. More research is needed to understand why this is the case, and how to improve the effects of technology-based CBT on quality of life.

DISCUSSION

There are several interesting avenues being pursued into technology-based CBT research, including determining when it works, for whom it works best, and for whom it is least effective. For example, interesting research is underway on how to best personalize treatment recommendations, and into stepped care models of delivering screening and treatment to people with depression, anxiety, and suicidal ideation. For example, the STAND project (Screening and Treatment for Anxiety and Depression at the University of California, Los Angeles, USA) includes digital screening and triages clients to levels of care based on their screening results. Levels of care include monitoring, digital CBT with coaching, digital CBT with clinician support, and clinical care with trained health professionals which included individually tailored CBT, pharmacotherapy, or both.[97] These studies will reveal the best way to tailor treatment recommendations to an individual's symptom severity.

Although this review has focused on technology-based CBT for treating mental disorders and symptoms, there is also interesting work testing the use of Internet CBT for loneliness,[98] as well as targeting transdiagnostic processes such as perfectionism[99,100] and rumination and worry.[101] These programs likely have broad appeal for those with or without mental health disorders.

Further research is needed on how to successfully adopt and integrate technology-supported CBT interventions into practice. Despite the evidence for technology-delivered CBT interventions, especially Internet CBT, barriers are still in place for their widespread use and uptake in routine mental health care settings. Barriers include clinician attitudes and concerns (eg, concerns about efficacy and safety), patient attitudes (eg, mistrust, concerns about data privacy), lack of training, and a lack of funding models to support blended and clinician-guided Internet CBT in practice. Implementation trials are needed to identify effective methods to successfully implement and sustain technology-based interventions in health care settings.

Although the most widely researched digital interventions are CBT, research also shows some promise for the use of third wave cognitive and behavioral therapies such as Internet Acceptance and Commitment Therapy,[102] mindfulness-based treatment approaches,[103,104] and short-term Internet psychodynamic therapy for depression.[105,106] This work will lead to better choice for patients, and evidence regarding the most effective treatment modality for different conditions.

Recent research has been examining the potential utility and efficacy of single-session brief technology interventions[107] and intensive Internet-intervention approaches[108,109] delivered online. These can speed up synchronous therapy time and may be suitable for people on wait lists or wanting shorter intensive treatment approaches.

A further area of future research involves the use of technology-based virtual reality (VR) approaches (see Ref[110] for an overview). Several reviews and meta-analyses of virtual reality exposure therapy have been published.[111] Virtual reality has clinical potential as a part of CBT, including use of virtual exposure scenarios that are impossible or impractical to do in session (eg, Ref[112]). Lindner[110] covers interesting future directions for the use of VR in therapy, including gamification, avatar therapists, virtual gatherings, and immersive storytelling. There is some emerging literature on treatments using immersive avatar therapy for psychosis, where a patient creates an avatar to represent their verbal auditory hallucinations, which can then be altered by the therapist in real-time as the patient interacts assertively with them.[113] These interventions may reduce the frequency of and even attenuate these hallucinations. Further research is needed in the effectiveness of VR interventions in real-world routine care settings and how they complement and augment CBT.

SUMMARY

Using technology to deliver CBT has several advantages of making treatment more accessible, convenient, and private, and overcoming barriers to care. Overall, there is well-established evidence for the use of Internet CBT for the treatment of depression and a range of anxiety and related disorders, and emerging evidence for Internet CBT in PTSD treatment. Evidence for the use of Internet CBT to treat other disorders such as eating disorders and substance-use disorders is inconclusive. There is some evidence that telehealth-delivered CBT is as effective as in-person CBT for depression and anxiety disorders, although again more research is needed for some disorders. Smartphone CBT apps for anxiety and depression appear to be effective but achieve smaller effect sizes than Internet-based CBT programs, and suffer from poor engagement when delivered as a standalone treatment without guidance. Overall technology provides an innovative way to disseminate CBT and reach more people who need effective treatment.

DISCLOSURE

J.M. Newby receives funding from the HCF Research Foundation, Australia, the Australian National Health and Medical Research Council (grant: 2008839), and Australian Medical Research Future Fund. These funding sources had no role in the content or the decision to publish this article.

REFERENCES

1. Newby J, Mason E, Kladnistki N, et al. Integrating internet CBT into clinical practice: a practical guide for clinicians. Clin Psychol 2021;25(2):164–78.
2. Andersson G, Carlbring P. Internet-assisted cognitive behavioral therapy. Psychiatric Clinics of North America 2017;40(4):689–700.
3. Kooistra LC, Wiersma JE, Ruwaard J, et al. Cost and Effectiveness of Blended Versus Standard Cognitive Behavioral Therapy for Outpatients With Depression

in Routine Specialized Mental Health Care: Pilot Randomized Controlled Trial. J Med Internet Res 2019;21(10):e14261.

4. Smith J, Newby JM, Burston N, et al. Help from home for depression: A randomised controlled trial comparing internet-delivered cognitive behaviour therapy with bibliotherapy for depression. Internet Interventions 2017;9:25–37.

5. Andrews G, Basu A, Cuijpers P, et al. Computer therapy for the anxiety and depression disorders is effective, acceptable and practical health care: An updated meta-analysis. J Anxiety Disord 2018;55:70–8.

6. Karyotaki E, Efthimiou O, Miguel C, et al. Internet-Based Cognitive Behavioral Therapy for Depression: A Systematic Review and Individual Patient Data Network Meta-analysis. JAMA Psychiatry 2021;78(4):361–71.

7. Newby JM, Twomey C, Yuan Li SS, et al. Transdiagnostic computerised cognitive behavioural therapy for depression and anxiety: A systematic review and meta-analysis. J Affect Disord 2016;199:30–41.

8. Hedman-Lagerlöf E, Carlbring P, Svärdman F, et al. Therapist-supported Internet-based cognitive behaviour therapy yields similar effects as face-to-face therapy for psychiatric and somatic disorders: an updated systematic review and meta-analysis. World Psychiatry 2023;22(2):305–14.

9. Luo C, Sanger N, Singhal N, et al. A comparison of electronically-delivered and face to face cognitive behavioural therapies in depressive disorders: A systematic review and meta-analysis. eClinicalMedicine 2020;24:100442.

10. Pauley D, Cuijpers P, Papola D, et al. Two decades of digital interventions for anxiety disorders: a systematic review and meta-analysis of treatment effectiveness. Psychol Med 2023;53(2):567–79.

11. Eilert N, Enrique A, Wogan R, et al. The effectiveness of Internet-delivered treatment for generalized anxiety disorder: An updated systematic review and meta-analysis. Depress Anxiety 2021;38(2):196–219.

12. Stech EP, Lim J, Upton EL, et al. Internet-delivered cognitive behavioral therapy for panic disorder with or without agoraphobia: a systematic review and meta-analysis. Cognit Behav Ther 2020;49(4):270–93.

13. Hedman E, Andersson G, Andersson E, et al. Internet-based cognitive-behavioural therapy for severe health anxiety: Randomised controlled trial. Br J Psychiatry 2011;198(3):230–6.

14. Machado-Sousa M, Moreira PS, Costa AD, et al. Efficacy of internet-based cognitive-behavioral therapy for obsessive-compulsive disorder: A systematic review and meta-analysis. Clin Psychol: Sci Pract 2023;30(2):150.

15. Dear BF, Staples LG, Terides MD, et al. Transdiagnostic versus disorder-specific and clinician-guided versus self-guided internet-delivered treatment for generalized anxiety disorder and comorbid disorders: A randomized controlled trial. J Anxiety Disord 2015;36:63–77.

16. Johnston L, Titov N, Andrews G, et al. A RCT of a transdiagnostic internet-delivered treatment for three anxiety disorders: examination of support roles and disorder-specific outcomes. PLoS One 2011;6(11):e28079.

17. Titov N, Dear BF, Staples LG, et al. Disorder-specific versus transdiagnostic and clinician-guided versus self-guided treatment for major depressive disorder and comorbid anxiety disorders: a randomized controlled trial. J Anxiety Disord 2015;35:88–102.

18. Guo S, Deng W, Wang H, et al. The efficacy of internet-based cognitive behavioural therapy for social anxiety disorder: A systematic review and meta-analysis. Clin Psychol Psychother 2021;28(3):656–68.

19. Aspvall K, Andersson E, Melin K, et al. Effect of an Internet-Delivered Stepped-Care Program vs In-Person Cognitive Behavioral Therapy on Obsessive-Compulsive Disorder Symptoms in Children and Adolescents: A Randomized Clinical Trial. JAMA 2021;325(18):1863–73.

20. Newby JM, Smith J, Uppal S, et al. Internet-based cognitive behavioural therapy versus psychoeducation control for illness anxiety disorder and somatic symptom disorder: a randomised controlled trial. J Consult Clin Psychol 2018;86(1):89–98.

21. Hedman E, Axelsson E, Andersson E, et al. Exposure-based cognitive–behavioural therapy via the internet and as bibliotherapy for somatic symptom disorder and illness anxiety disorder: randomised controlled trial. Br J Psychiatry 2016;209(5):407–13.

22. Hedman E, Axelsson E, Görling A, et al. Internet-delivered exposure-based cognitive-behavioural therapy and behavioural stress management for severe health anxiety: randomised controlled trial. Br J Psychiatry 2014;205(4):307–14.

23. Axelsson E, Andersson E, Ljótsson B, et al. Effect of Internet vs Face-to-Face Cognitive Behavior Therapy for Health Anxiety: A Randomized Noninferiority Clinical Trial. JAMA Psychiatry 2020;77(9):915–24.

24. Lewis C, Roberts NP, Simon N, et al. Internet-delivered cognitive behavioural therapy for post-traumatic stress disorder: systematic review and meta-analysis. Acta Psychiatr Scand 2019;140(6):508–21.

25. Zhou Y, Bai Z, Wu W, et al. Impacts of Internet-Based Interventions for Veterans With PTSD: A Systematic Review and Meta-Analysis. Front Psychol 2021;12:711652.

26. Ching H, Chua JYX, Chua JS, Shorey S. The effectiveness of technology-based cognitive behavioral therapy on perinatal depression and anxiety: A systematic review and meta-analysis. Worldviews Evid Based Nurs 2023;20(5):451–64.

27. Loughnan SA, Sie A, Hobbs MJ, et al. A randomized controlled trial of 'MUMentum Pregnancy': Internet-delivered cognitive behavioral therapy for antenatal anxiety and depression. J Affect Disord 2019;243:381–90.

28. Loughnan SA, Butler C, Sie AA, et al. A randomized controlled trial of 'MUMentum postnatal': Internet-delivered cognitive behavioural therapy for anxiety and depression in postpartum women. Behav Res Ther 2019;116:94–103.

29. Mu TY, Li YH, Xu RX, et al. Internet-based interventions for postpartum depression: A systematic review and meta-analysis. Nurs Open 2021;8(3):1125–34.

30. Newby JM, Robins L, Wilhelm K, et al. Web-based cognitive behavior therapy for depression in people with diabetes mellitus: A randomized controlled trial. J Med Internet Res 2017;19:e157.

31. Murphy MJ, Newby JM, Butow P, et al. Randomised controlled trial of internet-delivered cognitive behaviour therapy for clinical depression and/or anxiety in cancer survivors (iCanADAPT Early). Psycho Oncol 2020;29(1):76–85.

32. O'Moore K A, Newby JM, Andrews G, et al. Internet Cognitive-Behavioral Therapy for Depression in Older Adults With Knee Osteoarthritis: A Randomized Controlled Trial. Arthritis Care Res 2018;70(1):61–70.

33. Mehta S, Peynenburg VA, Hadjistavropoulos HD. Internet-delivered cognitive behaviour therapy for chronic health conditions: a systematic review and meta-analysis. J Behav Med 2019;42(2):169–87.

34. Cunnington D, Junge M. Chronic insomnia: diagnosis and non-pharmacological management. BMJ 2016;355:i5819.

35. Zachariae R, Lyby MS, Ritterband LM, et al. Efficacy of internet-delivered cognitive-behavioral therapy for insomnia - A systematic review and meta-analysis of randomized controlled trials. Sleep Med Rev 2016;30:1–10.

36. Soh HL, Ho RC, Ho CS, et al. Efficacy of digital cognitive behavioural therapy for insomnia: a meta-analysis of randomised controlled trials. Sleep Med 2020;75: 315–25.

37. Baka A, van der Zweerde T, Lancee J, et al. Cost-effectiveness of Guided Internet-Delivered Cognitive Behavioral Therapy in Comparison with Care-as-Usual for Patients with Insomnia in General Practice. Behav Sleep Med 2021; 20(2):188–203.

38. De Bruin EJ, van Steensel FJA, Meijer AM. Cost-Effectiveness of Group and Internet Cognitive Behavioral Therapy for Insomnia in Adolescents: Results from a Randomized Controlled Trial. Sleep 2016;39(8):1571–81.

39. Luik AI, Kyle SD, Espie CA. Digital Cognitive Behavioral Therapy (dCBT) for Insomnia: a State-of-the-Science Review. Current sleep medicine reports 2017;3(2):48–56.

40. Matthews EE, Arnedt JT, McCarthy MS, et al. Adherence to cognitive behavioral therapy for insomnia: a systematic review. Sleep Med Rev 2013;17(6):453–64.

41. Kalmbach DA, Cheng P, O'Brien LM, et al. A randomized controlled trial of digital cognitive behavioral therapy for insomnia in pregnant women. Sleep Med 2020;72:82–92.

42. Cheng P, et al. Digital cognitive behavioral therapy for insomnia promotes later health resilience during the coronavirus disease 19 (COVID-19) pandemic. Sleep 2021;44(4):zsab036.

43. Mason EC, Grierson AB, Sie A, et al. Co-occurring insomnia and anxiety: a randomized controlled trial of internet cognitive behavioral therapy for insomnia versus internet cognitive behavioral therapy for anxiety. Sleep 2023;46(2): zsac205.

44. Cheng P, Kalmbach DA, Tallent G, et al. Depression prevention via digital cognitive behavioral therapy for insomnia: a randomized controlled trial. Sleep 2019; 42(10):zsz150.

45. Moghimi E, Davis C, Rotondi M. The Efficacy of eHealth Interventions for the Treatment of Adults Diagnosed With Full or Subthreshold Binge Eating Disorder: Systematic Review and Meta-analysis. J Med Internet Res 2021;23(7):e17874.

46. Ahmadiankalati M, Steins-Loeber S, Paslakis G. Review of Randomized Controlled Trials Using e-Health Interventions for Patients With Eating Disorders. Front Psychiatry 2020;11:568.

47. de Zwaan M, Herpertz S, Zipfel S, et al. Effect of Internet-Based Guided Self-help vs Individual Face-to-Face Treatment on Full or Subsyndromal Binge Eating Disorder in Overweight or Obese Patients: The INTERBED Randomized Clinical Trial. JAMA Psychiatry 2017;74(10):987–95.

48. Zerwas SC, Watson HJ, Hofmeier SM, et al. CBT4BN: a randomized controlled trial of online chat and face-to-face group therapy for bulimia nervosa. Psychother Psychosom 2016;86(1):47–53.

49. Bonfiglio NS, Mascia ML, Cataudella S, et al. Digital Help for Substance Users (SU): A Systematic Review. Int J Environ Res Public Health 2022;19(18):11309.

50. Boumparis N, Loheide-Niesmann L, Blankers M, et al. Short- and long-term effects of digital prevention and treatment interventions for cannabis use reduction: A systematic review and meta-analysis. Drug Alcohol Depend 2019;200: 82–94.

51. Boumparis N, Karyotaki E, Schaub MP, et al. Internet interventions for adult illicit substance users: a meta-analysis. Addiction 2017;112(9):1521–32.

52. Hadjistavropoulos HD, Mehta S, Wilhelms A, et al. A systematic review of internet-delivered cognitive behavior therapy for alcohol misuse: study characteristics, program content and outcomes. Cognit Behav Ther 2020;49(4):327–46.

53. Boumparis N, Schulte MHJ, Riper H. Digital Mental Health for Alcohol and Substance Use Disorders. Current Treatment Options in Psychiatry 2019;6(4): 352–66.

54. Bellanti DM, Kelber MS, Workman DE, et al. Rapid Review on the Effectiveness of Telehealth Interventions for the Treatment of Behavioral Health Disorders. Mil Med 2022;187(5–6):e577–88.

55. Coughtrey AE, Pistrang N. The effectiveness of telephone-delivered psychological therapies for depression and anxiety: A systematic review. J Telemed Telecare 2018;24(2):65–74.

56. Berryhill MB, Culmer N, Williams N, et al. Videoconferencing Psychotherapy and Depression: A Systematic Review. Telemed J e Health 2019;25(6):435–46.

57. Mohr DC, Ho J, Duffecy J, et al. Effect of telephone-administered vs face-to-face cognitive behavioral therapy on adherence to therapy and depression outcomes among primary care patients: a randomized trial. JAMA 2012;307(21): 2278–85.

58. Kafali N, Cook B, Canino G, et al. Cost-effectiveness of a randomized trial to treat depression among Latinos. J Ment Health Pol Econ 2014;17(2):41–50.

59. Gentry MT, Lapid MI, Clark MM, et al. Evidence for telehealth group-based treatment: A systematic review. J Telemed Telecare 2019;25(6):327–42.

60. Komariah M, Amirah S, Faisal EG, et al. Efficacy of Internet-Based Cognitive Behavioral Therapy for Depression and Anxiety among Global Population during the COVID-19 Pandemic: A Systematic Review and Meta-Analysis of a Randomized Controlled Trial Study. Healthcare (Basel) 2022;10(7):1224.

61. Mahoney A, Li I, Grierson A, et al. Internet-based cognitive behaviour therapy for insomnia before and during the COVID-19 pandemic. Aust Psychol 2022; 57(1):65–76.

62. Mahoney AEJ, Elders A, Li I, et al. A tale of two countries: Increased uptake of digital mental health services during the COVID-19 pandemic in Australia and New Zealand. Internet Interventions 2021;25:100439.

63. Sharrock MJ, Mahoney AEJ, Haskelberg H, et al. The uptake and outcomes of Internet-based cognitive behavioural therapy for health anxiety symptoms during the COVID-19 pandemic. J Anxiety Disord 2021;84:102494.

64. Liu Z, Qiao D, Xu Y, et al. The Efficacy of Computerized Cognitive Behavioral Therapy for Depressive and Anxiety Symptoms in Patients With COVID-19: Randomized Controlled Trial. J Med Internet Res 2021;23(5):e26883.

65. Etzelmueller A, Vis C, Karyotaki E, et al. Effects of Internet-Based Cognitive Behavioral Therapy in Routine Care for Adults in Treatment for Depression and Anxiety: Systematic Review and Meta-Analysis. J Med Internet Res 2020; 22(8):e18100.

66. Niles AN, Axelsson E, Andersson E, et al. Internet-based cognitive behavior therapy for depression, social anxiety disorder, and panic disorder: Effectiveness and predictors of response in a teaching clinic. Behav Res Ther 2021; 136:103767.

67. Luu J, Millard M, Newby J, et al. Internet-based cognitive behavioural therapy for treating symptoms of obsessive compulsive disorder in routine care. Journal of Obsessive-Compulsive and Related Disorders 2020;26:100561.

68. Newby JM, Mackenzie A, Williams AD, et al. Internet cognitive behavioural therapy for mixed anxiety and depression: a randomized controlled trial and evidence of effectiveness in primary care. Psychol Med 2013;43(12):2635–48.
69. Haller K, Becker P, Niemeyer H, et al. Who benefits from guided internet-based interventions? A systematic review of predictors and moderators of treatment outcome. Internet Interv 2023;33:100635.
70. Reins JA, Buntrock C, Zimmermann J, et al. Efficacy and Moderators of Internet-Based Interventions in Adults with Subthreshold Depression: An Individual Participant Data Meta-Analysis of Randomized Controlled Trials. Psychother Psychosom 2021;90(2):94–106.
71. Furukawa TA, Suganuma A, Ostinelli EG, et al. Dismantling, optimising, and personalising internet cognitive behavioural therapy for depression: a systematic review and component network meta-analysis using individual participant data. Lancet Psychiatry 2021;8(6):500–11.
72. Musiat P, Johnson C, Atkinson M, et al. Impact of guidance on intervention adherence in computerised interventions for mental health problems: a meta-analysis. Psychol Med 2022;52(2):229–40.
73. Kaiser J, Hanschmidt F, Kersting A. The association between therapeutic alliance and outcome in internet-based psychological interventions: A meta-analysis. Comput Hum Behav 2021;114:106512.
74. Schmidt ID, Forand NR, Strunk DR. Predictors of Dropout in Internet-Based Cognitive Behavioral Therapy for Depression. Cognit Ther Res 2019;43(3): 620–30.
75. McCall HC, Hadjistavropoulos HD, Sundström CRF. Exploring the Role of Persuasive Design in Unguided Internet-Delivered Cognitive Behavioral Therapy for Depression and Anxiety Among Adults: Systematic Review, Meta-analysis, and Meta-regression. J Med Internet Res 2021;23(4):e26939.
76. Cheng VWS, Davenport T, Johnson D, et al. Gamification in Apps and Technologies for Improving Mental Health and Well-Being: Systematic Review. JMIR Ment Health 2019;6(6):e13717.
77. Six SG, Byrne KA, Tibbett TP, et al. Examining the Effectiveness of Gamification in Mental Health Apps for Depression: Systematic Review and Meta-analysis. JMIR Ment Health 2021;8(11):e32199.
78. Rozental A, Andersson G, Boettcher J, et al. Consensus statement on defining and measuring negative effects of Internet interventions. Internet Interventions 2014;1(1):12–9.
79. Rozental A, Magnusson K, Boettcher J, et al. For better or worse: An individual patient data meta-analysis of deterioration among participants receiving Internet-based cognitive behavior therapy. J Consult Clin Psychol 2017; 85(2):160.
80. Boettcher J, Rozental A, Andersson G, et al. Side effects in Internet-based interventions for social anxiety disorder. Internet Interventions 2014;1(1):3–11.
81. Marshall JM, Dunstan DA, Bartik W. Clinical or gimmickal: The use and effectiveness of mobile mental health apps for treating anxiety and depression. Aust N Z J Psychiatry 2020;54(1):20–8.
82. Lau N, O'Daffer A, Colt S, et al. Android and iPhone Mobile Apps for Psychosocial Wellness and Stress Management: Systematic Search in App Stores and Literature Review. JMIR Mhealth Uhealth 2020;8(5):e17798.
83. Eisenstadt M, Liverpool S, Infanti E, et al. Mobile Apps That Promote Emotion Regulation, Positive Mental Health, and Well-being in the General Population: Systematic Review and Meta-analysis. JMIR Ment Health 2021;8(11):e31170.

84. Anastasiadou D, Folkvord F, Lupiañez-Villanueva F. A systematic review of mHealth interventions for the support of eating disorders. Eur Eat Disord Rev 2018;26(5):394–416.

85. Goreis A, Felnhofer A, Kafka JX, et al. Efficacy of Self-Management Smartphone-Based Apps for Post-traumatic Stress Disorder Symptoms: A Systematic Review and Meta-Analysis. Front Neurosci 2020;14:3.

86. Firth J, Torous J, Nicholas J, et al. The efficacy of smartphone-based mental health interventions for depressive symptoms: a meta-analysis of randomized controlled trials. World Psychiatry 2017;16(3):287–98.

87. Lecomte T, Potvin S, Corbière M, et al. Mobile Apps for Mental Health Issues: Meta-Review of Meta-Analyses. JMIR Mhealth Uhealth 2020;8(5):e17458.

88. Firth J, Torous J, Nicholas J, et al. Can smartphone mental health interventions reduce symptoms of anxiety? A meta-analysis of randomized controlled trials. J Affect Disord 2017;218:15–22.

89. Huckvale K, Nicholas J, Torous J, et al. Smartphone apps for the treatment of mental health conditions: status and considerations. Current Opinion in Psychology 2020;36:65–70.

90. Torous J, Lipschitz J, Ng M, et al. Dropout rates in clinical trials of smartphone apps for depressive symptoms: A systematic review and meta-analysis. J Affect Disord 2020;263:413–9.

91. Melia R, Francis K, Hickey E, et al. Mobile Health Technology Interventions for Suicide Prevention: Systematic Review 2020;8(1):e12516.

92. Denecke K, Vaaheesan S, Arulnathan A. A Mental Health Chatbot for Regulating Emotions (SERMO) - Concept and Usability Test. IEEE Transactions on Emerging Topics in Computing 2021;9(3):1170–82.

93. Oh J, Jang S, Kim H, et al. Efficacy of mobile app-based interactive cognitive behavioral therapy using a chatbot for panic disorder. Int J Med Inf 2020;140:104171.

94. Martínez P, Rojas G, Martínez V, et al. Internet-based interventions for the prevention and treatment of depression in people living in developing countries: A systematic review. J Affect Disord 2018;234:193–200.

95. Spanhel K, Balci S, Feldhahn F, et al. Cultural adaptation of internet- and mobile-based interventions for mental disorders: a systematic review. npj Digital Medicine 2021;4(1):128.

96. Watfern C, Heck C, Rule C, et al. Feasibility and Acceptability of a Mental Health Website for Adults With an Intellectual Disability: Qualitative Evaluation. JMIR Ment Health 2019;6(3):e12958.

97. Wolitzky-Taylor K, LeBeau R, Arnaudova I, et al. A Novel and Integrated Digitally Supported System of Care for Depression and Anxiety: Findings From an Open Trial. JMIR Ment Health 2023;10:e46200.

98. Käll A, Bäck M, Welin C, et al. Therapist-Guided Internet-Based Treatments for Loneliness: A Randomized Controlled Three-Arm Trial Comparing Cognitive Behavioral Therapy and Interpersonal Psychotherapy. Psychother Psychosom 2021;90(5):351–8.

99. Wade TD, Kay E, de Valle MK, et al. Internet-based cognitive behaviour therapy for perfectionism: More is better but no need to be prescriptive. Clin Psychol 2019;23(3):196–205.

100. Rozental A, Shafran R, Wade TD, et al. Guided Web-Based Cognitive Behavior Therapy for Perfectionism: Results From Two Different Randomized Controlled Trials. J Med Internet Res 2018;20(4):e154.

101. Joubert AE, Grierson AB, Li I, et al. Managing Rumination and worry: A randomised controlled trial of an internet intervention targeting repetitive negative thinking delivered with and without clinician guidance. Behav Res Ther 2023; 168:104378.
102. Thompson EM, Destree L, Albertella L, et al. Internet-Based Acceptance and Commitment Therapy: A Transdiagnostic Systematic Review and Meta-Analysis for Mental Health Outcomes. Behav Ther 2021;52(2):492–507.
103. Boettcher J, Aström V, Påhlsson D, et al. Internet-Based Mindfulness Treatment for Anxiety Disorders: A Randomized Controlled Trial. Behav Ther 2014;45(2): 241–53.
104. Kladnitski N, Smith J, Uppal S, et al. Transdiagnostic internet-delivered CBT and mindfulness-based treatment for depression and anxiety: A randomised controlled trial. Internet Interventions 2020;20:100310.
105. Johansson R, Björklund M, Hornborg C, et al. Affect-focused psychodynamic psychotherapy for depression and anxiety through the Internet: a randomized controlled trial. PeerJ 2013;1:e102.
106. Johansson R, Ekbladh S, Hebert A, et al. Psychodynamic guided self-help for adult depression through the internet: A randomised controlled trial. PLoS One 2012;7(5):e38021.
107. Schleider JL, Mullarkey MC, Fox KR, et al. A randomized trial of online single-session interventions for adolescent depression during COVID-19. Nat Human Behav 2022;6(2):258–68.
108. Stech EP, Grierson AB, Chen AZ, et al. Intensive one-week internet-delivered cognitive behavioral therapy for panic disorder and agoraphobia: A pilot study. Internet Interv 2020;20:100315.
109. Jain N, Stech E, Grierson AB, et al. A pilot study of intensive 7-day internet-based cognitive behavioral therapy for social anxiety disorder. J Anxiety Disord 2021;84:102473.
110. Lindner P. Better, Virtually: the Past, Present, and Future of Virtual Reality Cognitive Behavior Therapy. Int J Cognit Ther 2021;14(1):23–46.
111. Freeman D, Reeve S, Robinson A, et al. Virtual reality in the assessment, understanding, and treatment of mental health disorders. Psychol Med 2017;47(14): 2393–400.
112. Jiang MYW, Upton E, Newby JM. A randomised wait-list controlled pilot trial of one-session virtual reality exposure therapy for blood-injection-injury phobias. J Affect Disord 2020;276:636–45.
113. du Sert OP, Potvin S, Lipp O, et al. Virtual reality therapy for refractory auditory verbal hallucinations in schizophrenia: A pilot clinical trial. Schizophr Res 2018; 197:176–81.

An Overview of Research on Acceptance and Commitment Therapy

Michael E. Levin, PhD[a],*, Jennifer Krafft, PhD[b],
Michael P. Twohig, PhD[a]

KEYWORDS

- Acceptance and commitment therapy • Mindfulness • Psychological flexibility
- Contextual behavioral science • Review

KEY POINTS

- Acceptance and commitment therapy (ACT) is a process-based treatment that has been applied widely to problem areas impacted by psychological inflexibility.
- Reviews of mediation research indicate that ACT improves outcomes by increasing psychological flexibility.
- Reviews of randomized controlled trials indicate the efficacy of ACT for depression, anxiety disorders, obsessive-compulsive and related disorders, psychosis, substance use disorders, chronic pain, coping with chronic health conditions, obesity, stigma, and stress and burnout.
- The evidence for ACT is growing in diverse cultural contexts, but more research is needed on ACT adapted and applied for minoritized and underserved populations.
- ACT is efficacious when applied through scalable, alternative treatment formats such as digital self-help and possibly when delivered by nonmental health professionals.

INTRODUCTION

Acceptance and commitment therapy (ACT)[1] is a modern cognitive behavioral therapy that has grown significantly in research and dissemination over the past 2 decades.[2] Although the methodological rigor of each trial varies, there are now well over 1000 randomized controlled trials (RCTs) on ACT for a wide range of areas across psychiatric conditions, chronic health conditions, and broader psychosocial concerns.[3] These RCTs represent efforts across the world in refining, studying, and delivering ACT, including in many countries outside of North America and Europe such as

[a] Department of Psychology, Utah State University, 2810 Old Main Hill, Logan, UT 84322, USA;
[b] Department of Psychology, Mississippi State University, 110 Magruder Hall, 255 Lee Boulevard, Mississippi State, MS 39762, USA
* Corresponding author.
E-mail address: Mike.Levin@usu.edu

Psychiatr Clin N Am 47 (2024) 419–431
https://doi.org/10.1016/j.psc.2024.02.007

Iran,[4] South Korea,[5] and countries throughout Sub-Saharan Africa,[6] among many others.[7] ACT has been increasingly adopted in empirically supported treatment guidelines throughout the world, such as the World Health Organization, the United Kingdom's National Institute for Health and Care Excellence, Australian Psychological Society, and American Psychological Association's Society of Clinical Psychology.[8]

In this article, we aim to provide an overarching summary of research on ACT as of 2023, with an emphasis on summarizing recent systematic reviews and meta-analytic evidence. This will include a brief summary of the conceptual foundations of ACT and the underlying psychological flexibility model, followed by a review of treatment outcome research.

CONCEPTUAL FOUNDATIONS OF ACCEPTANCE AND COMMITMENT THERAPY

The defining features of ACT are rooted in its conceptual foundations, beginning with functional contextualism as the underlying philosophy of science.[9] Functional contextualism diverges from the dominant perspective of science, which is to model the world as it *truly* is, by instead defining the analytical goals of science in terms of what works to predict and influence behavior. A core assumption is that behavior can only be understood (ie, predicted and influenced) in context, and thus methods and constructs are emphasized that examine the relations between behavior and context. To better clarify the unique assumptions and implications of functional contextualism for research, contextual behavioral science[10] (CBS) is used to describe the research paradigm underlying ACT, among other areas of scholarship rooted in this philosophy of science. CBS employs a reticulated strategy to theory building and testing that integrates the areas of basic science, including behavior analysis and relational frame theory (RFT),[11] with applied treatment research.

RFT highlights how human's capacity to arbitrarily derive relations between stimuli, and to alter the function of those stimuli due to these relations, is a core feature of how cognition works in adaptive and maladaptive ways. For example, thinking "If I look anxious, then people will laugh at me" involves a series of relations (eg, "if-then," "I-others") that if responded to in a literal context (ie, perceiving thoughts as true) could lead to sensations like one's heartbeat being experienced as threatening and eliciting more anxiety. Consistent with the focus on context, RFT also suggests that the context of these relations could be altered such that this could be responded to as just a thought ("*I'm having the thought that* if I look anxious, then people will laugh at me"), which might change how it functions, such as by reducing the experience of one's heartbeat as threatening and anxiety eliciting. Altering the function of inner experiences over their content is a key focus of ACT and is informed by RFT.

THE PSYCHOLOGICAL FLEXIBILITY MODEL

ACT theorizes that *psychological inflexibility* is the core process in the development and maintenance of psychopathology: a pattern of behavior in which rigid responses to internal stimuli dominate, rather than personal values and direct contingencies, in influencing actions.[12] Subprocesses that contribute to psychological inflexibility include maladaptive responses to internal experiences such as experiential avoidance (ie, rigid patterns of behavior focused on avoiding or otherwise altering one's internal experience), cognitive fusion (ie, interacting with the content of thoughts on a literal basis such that they rigidly influence behavior), and attachment to a conceptualized self (ie, overly engaging with a rigid, cognitively fused sense of self).

A large body of research supports the relevance of psychological inflexibility to psychological problems. One recent meta-analysis of 441 studies found experiential avoidance to have moderate-to-large relations ($r = .34–.56$) with anxiety, depression, panic, obsessive-compulsive and related disorders (OCRDs), and post-traumatic stress disorder.[13] Another meta-analysis of 72 studies found deficits in valued action had medium-to-large relations with anxiety ($r = .26$) and depression ($r = .42$).[14] A meta-analysis of 181 studies assessing emotion regulation in youth found that avoidance had medium-to-large positive relations with depression, anxiety, and addiction ($r = .30–.46$), while acceptance had medium-to-large negative relations with these outcomes ($r = .23–.42$).[15]

Psychological inflexibility is targeted in ACT by increasing *psychological flexibility,* the ability to engage in valued patterns of activity while accepting whatever internal experiences arise. Psychological flexibility is composed of subprocesses that directly target maladaptive inflexible responses to internal experiences including cognitive defusion (ie, responding to thoughts as just thoughts), self-as-context (ie, experiencing a sense of self distinct from verbal labels), and acceptance of internal experiences. Psychological flexibility also includes subprocesses that further leverage the adaptive functions of cognition including clarifying personal values, committed action (ie, consistent patterns of behavior in pursuit of values), and flexible attention to the present moment.

As a process-focused treatment, ACT is applied broadly to any problem areas where psychological inflexibility plays a key role and/or psychological flexibility can lead to improvements. The specific protocols vary based on the population and treatment setting in terms of how psychological flexibility is targeted (eg, treatment length, exercises used), but share the process-based emphasis on psychological flexibility.

Consistent with the philosophy underlying ACT, the aim of the psychological flexibility model is not merely to accurately predict psychopathology, but to help influence change in the form needed for the client. Meta-analyses indicate that ACT is efficacious in reducing psychological inflexibility and increasing psychological flexibility across problem areas.[2,16–19] More importantly, mediation research supports the theory that ACT improves outcomes for clients by enhancing psychological flexibility. One meta-analysis of 50 ACT mediation studies found that increases in overall psychological flexibility, as well as subprocesses including acceptance, contact with the present moment, and values, significantly mediated treatment outcomes.[20] A meta-analysis of ACT for pain found that changes in pain acceptance and psychological flexibility mediated changes in disability.[21] Another meta-analysis found across 10 RCTs that the effects of ACT for anxiety and depression were significantly mediated by changes in psychological flexibility processes ($r = .16$).[22]

REVIEWS OF RANDOMIZED CONTROLLED TRIALS

The following sections review the evidence for RCTs evaluating ACT using recent (as of 2023) meta-analyses and systematic reviews. Areas are included in this review that have significant evidence bases for ACT, as indicated by reviews published in the past few years that can reasonably draw at least tentative conclusions on the available research.

Depression

The first RCT ever completed on ACT was for depression, which sought to examine whether depressive cognitions could be addressed with defusion and acceptance rather than cognitive restructuring.[23] Since then, substantial work has occurred in ACT for depression. A meta-analysis of 55 RCTs found ACT to be superior to inactive and weaker active controls like treatment-as-usual (TAU) for depression.[24] This meta-analysis found an advantage for CBT over ACT on depression at post-treatment

($d = -0.52$), but this was not present at follow-up ($d = -0.14$).[24] However, other reviews and meta-analyses have generally found equivalent efficacy for ACT and other CBTs for depression.[2,16] Another meta-analysis of 40 RCTs evaluating group-based ACT found significant effects on depression favoring ACT relative to inactive ($g = .55$) and active control conditions ($g = .30$).[25]

Anxiety and Anxiety Disorders

While the work in ACT is minor compared to the vast literature in exposure-based CBTs, there are supportive studies of ACT for each major anxiety disorder specifically as well as transdiagnostic protocols applied across anxiety disorders.[16] An umbrella review of systematic reviews and meta-analyses found 14 meta-analyses and 11 systematic reviews on ACT for anxiety and depression, with the majority of these studies being on anxiety.[16] Results support ACT over passive and active control conditions, with the exception being CBTs where no difference is found between ACT and other CBTs.[16] A meta-analysis of 12 RCTs evaluating ACT specifically for participants with anxiety disorders found significant effects favoring ACT to TAU on clinician-rated (standardized mean difference [SMD] = .98) and participant-rated anxiety (SMD = .99), but no significant difference between ACT and other CBTs.[26] A meta-analysis of 34 RCTs evaluating group-based ACT more broadly with any study that measured anxiety as an outcome found a medium effect favoring ACT to inactive control conditions ($g = .70$) but a nonsignificant small effect relative to active control conditions including CBT ($g = .17$).[25] In summary, ACT appears to be a viable treatment of anxiety issues, which might be particularly considered when CBT is not effective or when the clinical conditions suggest ACT is a better match.

Obsessive-compulsive and Related Disorders

Recent reviews and meta-analyses of ACT for obsessive-compulsive disorder (OCD) have identified more than 20 RCTs and repeatedly found that protocols containing ACT without in-session exposure and with in-session exposure work equivalently to other empirically supported treatments such as exposure with response prevention or a more traditional CBT protocol.[4,27] In a recent meta-analysis of ACT for OCD, an SMD of -1.19 was found in favor of ACT over control conditions,[27] but like the other recent reviews,[4] there is a significant variability in these ACT studies across many variables.

Work in OCD-related disorders such as body dysmorphic disorder, Tourette's disorder, chronic skin picking disorder, and hoarding disorder is just beginning, but each area has some research completed.[28] A fairly substantial line of research has occurred for trichotillomania using a combination of stimulus control, habit reversal, and ACT called ACT-enhanced behavior therapy (A-EBT). To date, there have been 6 RCTs on A-EBT in addition to a few open trials and single-subject designs.[28] A-EBT compared to waitlists has been shown to be effective in person, via telehealth, and over an asynchronous Web-based program.[28] In the largest trial to date ($N = 78$), A-EBT versus supportive psychotherapy showed 48% responder status in ACT and 28% in the active control condition.[29] Overall, these results suggest that ACT for OCD and A-EBT for trichotillomania have notable empirical support, while evidence is preliminary for ACT as a treatment for other OCRDs.

Psychosis

The psychosocial treatment of psychosis varies from many other diagnostic categories in that reduction in certain symptoms of the disorder is secondary to improving functioning. Thus, Acceptance and Commitment Therapy for Psychosis (ACTp) has an equal, if not stronger, focus on quality of life and functioning over reduction in psychosis. Recent meta-analyses of ACTp often combine it with other mindfulness therapies. Morris and colleagues recently reviewed these meta-analyses and found that ACTp is "safe and efficacious across a range of clinical outcomes and processes, including psychotic symptoms, depression, anxiety, functioning, help-seeking, satisfaction, rehospitalization reduction, mindfulness and psychological flexibility."[30] This review included 4 meta-analyses of ACTp specifically (with 4–8 RCTs included in each meta-analysis), finding significant effects favoring ACTp for reducing positive symptoms (SMD = .63), negative symptoms (SMD = .65), affective symptoms (SMD = .63–.64), and rehospitalization (odds ratio = .37–.41; risk ratio = .54).[30] Thus, ACTp appears to be efficacious in helping reduce symptoms associated with psychosis and increasing functioning.

Substance Use Disorders

Cigarette smoking has been one of the earliest and most established areas of ACT research. A meta-analysis of 19 RCTs across 6 countries found greater cessation rates for ACT relative to control conditions at follow-up (risk ratio = 1.70–1.80).[31] There has been less research on other substance use disorders, but preliminary results are promising.[32] A meta-analysis in 2015 largely captures the available RCT evidence to date, finding across 5 RCTs that ACT led to greater cessation of drug use compared to active control conditions at post-treatment (g = .45).[33]

Chronic Pain

There is a well-established literature indicating the efficacy of ACT for chronic pain, primarily relative to TAU, placebo, or no treatment comparison conditions. A meta-analysis of 33 RCTs with adult chronic pain patients found significant small-to-medium effect sizes favoring ACT relative to control conditions (waitlist, TAU, placebo) on physical functioning (g = .59), pain intensity (g = .44), and depression, anxiety, and quality of life (g = .43).[34] Moderation analyses indicated smaller, but still significant, effect sizes for longer (6–12 month) follow-up time points, nonspecific and mixed pain samples, and digital interventions relative to face-to-face therapy.[34]

Chronic Health Conditions

ACT has been applied to improve quality of life across a wide range of chronic health conditions. In a meta-analysis of 55 RCTs and quasi-experimental studies, the most frequent studies were conducted among patients with cancer (n = 35) and diabetes (n = 9), with other studies including patients with overweight (n = 4), stroke (n = 3), coronary heart disease (n = 2), epilepsy (n = 2), asthma (n = 1), and arthritis (n = 1).[35] Significant medium-to-large effect sizes were found favoring ACT to comparison conditions on quality of life (SMD = .87) and symptom improvement (SMD = .77), including relative to active treatment comparisons specifically (quality of life SMD = .79; symptoms SMD = .53).[35] Preliminary, but more mixed, results were found for ACT in improving quality of life and depression/anxiety symptoms among patients with multiple sclerosis in a review that included 5 RCTs.[36] A review of 10 RCTs evaluating ACT or other mindfulness-based treatments for inflammatory bowel disease found small effect sizes for improving quality of life and mental health relative to control conditions (SMD = .15–.39), but no effects on disease activity.[37]

Studies have found ACT improves disease management for some chronic health conditions. A review of ACT RCTs conducted specifically in Iran found that ACT significantly improved HbA1c in 7 of 9 studies and blood pressure in 5 studies.[4] A review of ACT for patients with cardiovascular disease found that ACT improved self-management of cardiovascular disease in 5 RCTs (eg, adherence to treatment recommendations, physical activity, self-care skills).[38] A review of 3 RCTs found ACT significantly improved impairment related to tinnitus.[39] Compared to TAU, ACT was found to improve initiation of antiretroviral treatment and engagement in substance use treatment in a sample of 100 participants with HIV using injection drugs.[40] ACT has also been used to increase health behaviors in various samples. For example, a meta-analysis of 5 RCTs found a significant small effect size favoring ACT to control conditions on increasing physical activity (SMD = .32).[41]

Obesity

ACT has been used with individuals with overweight to focus on addressing outcomes including weight loss, health behaviors, weight self-stigma, and/or quality of life. A systematic review of 16 RCTs found positive, though somewhat mixed, evidence for ACT in targeting these outcomes, with the results varying based on the outcomes targeted, the intensity of the ACT intervention, the rigor and follow-up length of assessments, and the comparison condition, which range from no treatment controls to standard behavior therapy.[42] A meta-analysis that combined these heterogeneous studies found a significant medium effect favoring ACT on body mass index (weighted mean difference [WMD] = .50) and weight self-stigma across 5 RCTs (WMD = .77) but with nonsignificant small effects for eating behaviors and quality of life.[17]

Stigma

One review identified 12 RCTs evaluating ACT for self-stigma and shame in a range of populations including individuals with psychiatric disorders, substance use disorders, and overweight.[43] Although there were some mixed results across studies, overall these RCTs tended to find ACT-reduced self-stigma and shame while improving quality of life and mental health. Another review found in 7 studies (combining RCTs, quasi-experimental, and single-arm designs) that ACT significantly improved stigma toward others (primarily individuals with psychiatric conditions, with one study evaluating ACT to reduce racial prejudice).[44]

Stress and Burnout

ACT has been applied in target populations experiencing stress and burnout. A meta-analysis of 10 RCTs evaluating ACT for health care workers found significant small effect sizes for work-related burnout and stress at follow-up relative to inactive (g = .25) and active comparison conditions (g = .36), but these effects were not present at posttreatment.[45] Another meta-analysis of 17 RCTs evaluating ACT in the workplace found a significant medium effect size for reducing distress relative to active and inactive control conditions among non-health care workers (8 RCTs; g = .51), but a nonsignificant small effect size for health care workers (9 RCTs; g = .22).[19]

ACT has also been studied for family caregivers. A meta-analysis of 7 RCTs with parents caregiving for a child with autism or a chronic health condition found significant small-to-medium effects favoring ACT relative to active and inactive control conditions on measures of distress (SMD = .55) and parenting confidence (SMD = .34).[46] Another meta-analysis of 11 RCTs combining caregivers of adults or children with chronic health conditions found significant small-to-medium effects favoring ACT to TAU/placebo control conditions on depression (SMD = .46), anxiety (SMD = .30), and stress (SMD = .54).[47]

Children and Adolescents

A review identified 34 studies (including case studies, single-case designs, single-arm trials, and 13 RCTs) evaluating ACT for children and adolescents.[48] Although the results are largely based on small pilot trials, initial findings suggest ACT might similarly be effective with children and adolescents for chronic pain, anxiety, OCRDs, depression, conduct problems, and eating disorders. A meta-analysis of 14 RCTs evaluating ACT with children (published in English or Chinese) found significant large effects favoring ACT to waitlist on depression and anxiety (SMD = .86) and quality of life (SMD = 1.74) as well as a medium effect favoring ACT to TAU on depression and anxiety (SMD = .59), but not for quality of life compared to TAU.[49] ACT was found to be equivalent to CBT in the 4 RCTs comparing these active treatments with children.[49]

Diverse Populations

Although ACT shares the common problem among other psychotherapies of being overly developed in and based on populations that are Western, Educated, Industrialized, Rich, and Democratic (WEIRD), there are growing bodies of evidence for ACT in non-WEIRD populations. Most notably, a review identified 110 RCTs that provide empirical support for ACT in Iran across a wide range of mental health concerns.[4] Another review identified 59 RCTs and quasi-experimental studies generally indicating empirical support for ACT in South Korea for a wide range of outcomes.[5] A review on ACT in Sub-Saharan Africa found 8 RCTs and single-arm trials, which generally provided support for the efficacy of ACT in targeting a range of mental health outcomes.[6] These examples highlight the breadth and depth of ACT research occurring outside of non-WEIRD populations to further evaluate, adapt, and refine ACT for diverse populations.

The representation of racial, sexual, and gender minorities in ACT trials is generally limited overall, and further research is needed to determine the generalizability and adaptation needs of ACT for minoritized populations.[50] Preliminary research has been conducted, for example, in LGBTQI+ populations, with a review of 5 studies on ACT with LGBTQI+ individuals finding ACT buffered the impact of proximal and distal minority stressors and improved mental health and quality of life, but much more research is needed.[51]

Alternate Treatment Delivery Methods

Similar to trends in CBT more broadly, a large body of research has developed over the past decade indicating ACT can be effectively delivered in digital, self-guided formats (ie, self-help Web sites and mobile apps) for a wide range of populations and problem areas. A meta-analysis of 53 RCTs evaluating ACT in Web or app formats found significant small effects favoring ACT to waitlist on anxiety ($g = .30$), depression ($g = .44$), and quality of life ($g = .20$), with more mixed results for active control group comparisons.[18]

Another strategy to increase reach and access to ACT is by training individuals who are not mental health professionals to deliver the intervention. A review identified 17 studies (10 of which were completed RCTs) evaluating ACT delivered by nonmental health professionals and community members including other health care workers, teachers, students, mothers, correctional staff, and other community adults.[52] Results indicated 16 of 17 studies found promising, positive results for ACT delivered by nonmental health professionals and community members for participants with mental health concerns, chronic health conditions, and caregivers.[52]

DISCUSSION

This review highlights the breadth and scope of ACT outcome research across varied psychiatric and chronic health conditions as well as addressing broader psychosocial concerns. Overall, the existing RCT evidence base indicates ACT can be applied to effectively treat a broad range of problem areas, including alternative, scalable formats such as digital self-help and when delivered by nonmental health professionals. This work has been conducted in diverse populations throughout the world, indicating that ACT can be adapted and implemented in other cultural contexts, although more work is needed in studying ACT with minoritized and underserved populations. Importantly, research also supports the underlying theoretic model ACT is based on, with changes in psychological flexibility accounting for how ACT improves these mental health outcomes.

Several limitations should be noted when considering the evidence base for ACT. As noted previously, much more research is needed on ACT in non-WEIRD populations and among people with minoritized identities. Additionally, many of the meta-analyses in this review identified concerns with methodological quality in some of the included RCTs,[4,5,17,25,26,42,43,45,49] including small sample sizes, handling of missing data, lack of masking, questionable randomization practices, problems with representativeness of samples, lack of assessor training, and lack of power analysis. Limitations related to measurement are also notable. From a theoretic perspective, the primary aim of ACT is to increase valued living, rather than reduce negatively evaluated inner experiences[12]; however, valued living is rarely the primary outcome in ACT treatment trials,[2] creating a discrepancy between the model and research base. Measurement of ACT treatment processes has also relied heavily on one self-report measure with notable conceptual and psychometric limitations, and mediational research would be strengthened through the use of alternative ACT process measures.[53]

Although ACT has been evaluated with just about any major problem area that might be treated by a psychosocial intervention, the strength of evidence for ACT varies. This review focused on more developed areas of ACT research. That said, there are other areas that have multiple positive RCTs and/or single-arm trials that were not reviewed including eating disorders,[54] post-traumatic stress disorder,[55] insomnia,[56] intimate partner violence,[57] and adults with autism or intellectual disabilities,[58] among other areas.

Another limitation of this review is the focus on RCTs for targeted conditions. This approach to categorizing evidence for ACT based on diagnostic categories and evaluating efficacy using group-level averages misses key information from a process-based therapy perspective, which ultimately is focused on clinical decision-making for individual clients.[59] In the future, more research is needed that examines idiographic patterns of change to see who specifically benefits from treatment, and how, which can then be scaled back up to nomothetic information that guides clinical decision-making.[59] The effect of averaging change across individuals, categorized by topographically defined syndromes, is a likely contributor to the lack of clear information in the literature on which treatment will be more beneficial to which clients (eg, when should I use ACT or cognitive therapy or behavioral activation for this problem?). Rather than "horse race" tests that have a "winner take all" approach in testing superior efficacy across an average of all people in a diagnostic category, more research is needed that drills down to understand which therapeutic processes are more beneficial to target, how, and for whom. One of our hopes in this review is that by highlighting the existing RCT evidence for ACT, the field can increasingly become empowered and motivated to move beyond testing the broad questions of the efficacy of ACT for particular conditions to these more precise, innovative areas of discovery needed to guide the more specific challenges faced in clinical decision-making.

SUMMARY

Consistent with the process-based approach, ACT is efficacious for a wide range of problem areas to which psychological flexibility applies. Although the strength of the evidence base varies across these areas, the research continues to grow rapidly and with increasingly rigorous trials being conducted in specific populations.

CLINICS CARE POINTS

- Consider conceptualizing clients' presenting concerns in terms of how and where psychological inflexibility is contributing and how psychological flexibility could produce meaningful changes.
- Although randomized controlled trials for specific conditions often focus on changes in symptoms, it is important to remember the goal of acceptance and commitment therapy (ACT) is to increase valued living (ie, engaging in what matters to clients, even when difficult internal experiences arise).
- ACT has been found efficacious for a wide range of mental health concerns, but there is not clear evidence of superior efficacy in most areas over other well-established cognitive behavioral therapies, so consider evidence-based practice principles in deciding which treatment is the best fit for a given client. Also, routine outcome monitoring is always important to assess whether treatment is working for your individual client.

DISCLOSURE

The authors have nothing to disclose.

REFERENCES

1. Hayes SC, Strosahl K, Wilson KG. Acceptance and Commitment therapy: the process and practice of mindful change. 2nd edition. New York, NY: Guilford Press; 2012.
2. Gloster AT, Walder N, Levin ME, et al. The empirical status of acceptance and commitment therapy: A review of meta-analyses. J Context Behav Sci 2020;18: 181–92.
3. Association for Contextual Behavioral Science. ACT Randomized Controlled Trials (1986 to present). 2023. https://contextualscience.org/act_randomized_controlled_trials_1986_to_present.
4. Akbari M, Seydavi M, Davis CH, et al. The current status of acceptance and commitment therapy (ACT) in Iran: A systematic narrative review. J Context Behav Sci 2022;26:85–96.
5. An W. A systematic review and meta-analysis of acceptance and commitment therapy in South Korea. Logan, UT: Utah State University; 2020.
6. Geda YE, Krell-Roesch J, Fisseha Y, et al. Acceptance and commitment therapy in a low-income country in sub-Saharan Africa: a call for further research. Front Public Health 2021;9:732800.
7. Association for Contextual Behavioral Science. ACT studies in Low and Middle Income Countries. 2023. https://contextualscience.org/act_studies_in_low_and_middle_income_countries.
8. Association for Contextual Behavioral Science. State of the ACT Evidence. 2023. https://contextualscience.org/state_of_the_act_evidence.

9. Hayes SC, Hayes LJ, Reese HW. Finding the philosophical core: A review of Stephen C. Pepper's World Hypotheses: A Study in Evidence. J Exp Anal Behav 1988;50(1):97.

10. Hayes SC, Barnes-Holmes D, Wilson KG. Contextual behavioral science: Creating a science more adequate to the challenge of the human condition. J Context Behav Sci 2012;1(1–2):1–16.

11. Hayes SC, Barnes-Holmes D, Roche B. Relational frame theory: a post-skinnerian account of human language and cognition. New York, NY: Kluwer; 2001.

12. Hayes SC, Levin ME, Plumb-Vilardaga J, et al. Acceptance and commitment therapy and contextual behavioral science: Examining the progress of a distinctive model of behavioral and cognitive therapy. Behav Ther 2013;44:180–98. https://doi.org/10.1016/j.beth.2009.08.002.

13. Akbari M, Seydavi M, Hosseini ZS, et al. Experiential avoidance in depression, anxiety, obsessive-compulsive related, and posttraumatic stress disorders: A comprehensive systematic review and meta-analysis. J Context Behav Sci 2022;24:65–78.

14. Tunç H, Morris PG, Kyranides MN, et al. The relationships between valued living and depression and anxiety: A systematic review, meta-analysis, and meta-regression. J Context Behav Sci 2023;28:102–26.

15. Kraft L, Ebner C, Leo K, et al. Emotion regulation strategies and symptoms of depression, anxiety, aggression, and addiction in children and adolescents: A meta-analysis and systematic review. Clin Psychol Sci Pract 2023;30(4):485–502.

16. Beygi Z, Jangali RT, Derakhshan N, et al. An overview of reviews on the effects of acceptance and commitment therapy (ACT) on depression and anxiety. Iran J Psychiatry 2023;18(2):248–57.

17. Chew HSJ, Chng S, Rajasegaran NN, et al. Effectiveness of acceptance and commitment therapy on weight, eating behaviours and psychological outcomes: a systematic review and meta-analysis. Eat Weight Disord-Stud Anorex Bulim Obes 2023;28(1):6.

18. Klimczak KS, San Miguel GG, Mukasa MN, et al. A systematic review and meta-analysis of self-guided online acceptance and commitment therapy as a transdiagnostic self-help intervention. Cognit Behav Ther 2023;52(3):269–94.

19. Unruh I, Neubert M, Wilhelm M, et al. ACT in the workplace: A meta-analytic examination of randomized controlled trials. J Context Behav Sci 2022;26:114–24.

20. Ren Z, Zhao C, Bian C, et al. Mechanisms of the acceptance and commitment therapy: A meta-analytic structural equation model. Acta Psychol Sin 2019;51(6):662–76.

21. Murillo C, Vo TT, Vansteelandt S, et al. How do psychologically based interventions for chronic musculoskeletal pain work? A systematic review and meta-analysis of specific moderators and mediators of treatment. Clin Psychol Rev 2022;94:102160.

22. Johannsen M, Nissen ER, Lundorff M, et al. Mediators of acceptance and mindfulness-based therapies for anxiety and depression: A systematic review and meta-analysis. Clin Psychol Rev 2022;94:102156.

23. Zettle RD, Hayes SC. Dysfunctional control by client verbal behavior: The context of reason-giving. Anal Verbal Behav 1986;4:30–8.

24. Williams AJ, Botanov Y, Giovanetti AK, et al. A metascientific review of the evidential value of acceptance and commitment therapy for depression. Behav Ther 2022;54(6):989–1005.

25. Ferreira MG, Mariano LI, de Rezende JV, et al. Effects of group Acceptance and Commitment Therapy (ACT) on anxiety and depressive symptoms in adults: A meta-analysis. J Affect Disord 2022;309:297–308.
26. Haller H, Breilmann P, Schröter M, et al. A systematic review and meta-analysis of acceptance-and mindfulness-based interventions for DSM-5 anxiety disorders. Sci Rep 2021;11(1):20385.
27. Soondrum T, Wang X, Gao F, et al. The applicability of acceptance and commitment therapy for obsessive-compulsive disorder: A systematic review and meta-analysis. Brain Sci 2022;12(5):656.
28. Krafft J, Petersen JM, Twohig M. Acceptance and commitment therapy for obsessive-compulsive and related disorders. In: Storch EA, Abramowitz JS, McKay D, editors. *Complexities in obsessive compulsive and related disorders: advances in conceptualization and treatment*. Oxford, UK: Oxford University Press; 2021. p. 352–C19.P98.
29. Woods DW, Ely LJ, Bauer CC, et al. Acceptance-enhanced behavior therapy for trichotillomania in adults: A randomized clinical trial. Behav Res Ther 2022;158: 104187.
30. Morris EM, Johns LC, Gaudiano BA. Acceptance and commitment therapy for psychosis: Current status, lingering questions and future directions. Psychol Psychother Theor Res Pract 2023;97(1):41–58.
31. Kwan YK, Lau Y, Ang WW, et al. Immediate, short-term, medium-term, and long-term effects of acceptance and commitment therapy for smoking cessation: a systematic review and meta-analysis. Nicotine Tob Res 2023;26(1):12–22.
32. Balandeh E, Omidi A, Ghaderi A. A narrative review of third-wave cognitive-behavioral therapies in addiction. Addict Health 2021;13(1):52.
33. Lee EB, An W, Levin ME, et al. An initial meta-analysis of acceptance and commitment therapy for treating substance use disorders. Drug Alcohol Depend 2015; 155:1–7.
34. Lai L, Liu Y, McCracken I M, et al. The efficacy of acceptance and commitment therapy for chronic pain: A three-level meta-analysis and a trial sequential analysis of randomized controlled trials. Behav Res Ther 2023;165:104308.
35. Konstantinou P, Ioannou M, Melanthiou D, et al. The impact of acceptance and commitment therapy (ACT) on quality of life and symptom improvement among chronic health conditions: A systematic review and meta-analysis. J Context Behav Sci 2023;29:240–53.
36. Zarotti N, Eccles F, Broyd A, et al. Third wave cognitive behavioural therapies for people with multiple sclerosis: a scoping review. Disabil Rehabil 2023;45(10): 1720–35.
37. Riggott C, Mikocka-Walus A, Gracie DJ, et al. Efficacy of psychological therapies in people with inflammatory bowel disease: a systematic review and meta-analysis. Lancet Gastroenterol Hepatol 2023;8(10):919–31.
38. Zhang X, Haixia M, Yee LC, et al. Effectiveness of acceptance and commitment therapy on self-care, psychological symptoms, and quality of life in patients with cardiovascular disease: a systematic review and meta-analysis. J Context Behav Sci 2023;29:46–58.
39. Ungar OJ, Handzel O, Abu Eta R, et al. Meta-analysis of acceptance and commitment therapy for tinnitus. Indian J Otolaryngol Head Neck Surg 2023;75(4): 2921–6.
40. Luoma JB, Rossi SL, Sereda Y, et al. An acceptance-based, intersectional stigma coping intervention for people with HIV who inject drugs—a randomized clinical trial. Lancet Reg Heal 2023;28:100611.

41. Pears S, Sutton S. Effectiveness of Acceptance and Commitment Therapy (ACT) interventions for promoting physical activity: a systematic review and meta-analysis. Health Psychol Rev 2021;15(1):159–84.

42. Iturbe I, Echeburúa E, Maiz E. The effectiveness of acceptance and commitment therapy upon weight management and psychological well-being of adults with overweight or obesity: A systematic review. Clin Psychol Psychother 2022; 29(3):837–56.

43. Stynes G, Leão CS, McHugh L. Exploring the effectiveness of mindfulness-based and third wave interventions in addressing self-stigma, shame and their impacts on psychosocial functioning: a systematic review. J Context Behav Sci 2022;23: 174–89.

44. Krafft J, Ferrell J, Levin ME, et al. Psychological inflexibility and stigma: A meta-analytic review. J Context Behav Sci 2018;7:15–28.

45. Prudenzi A, Graham CD, Clancy F, et al. Group-based acceptance and commitment therapy interventions for improving general distress and work-related distress in healthcare professionals: A systematic review and meta-analysis. J Affect Disord 2021;295:192–202.

46. Wright SR, Graham CD, Houghton R, et al. Acceptance and commitment therapy (ACT) for caregivers of children with chronic conditions: A mixed methods systematic review (MMSR) of efficacy, process, and acceptance. J Context Behav Sci 2023;27:72–97.

47. Han A, Yuen HK, Jenkins J. Acceptance and commitment therapy for family caregivers: A systematic review and meta-analysis. J Health Psychol 2021;26(1): 82–102.

48. Petersen JM, Ona PZ, Twohig MP. A review of acceptance and commitment therapy for adolescents: developmental and contextual considerations. Cogn Behav Pract 2024;31:72–89.

49. Fang S, Ding D. A meta-analysis of the efficacy of acceptance and commitment therapy for children. J Context Behav Sci 2020;15:225–34.

50. Misra A, Bryan A, Faber NS, et al. A systematic review of inclusion of minoritized populations in randomized controlled trials of acceptance and commitment therapy. J Context Behav Sci 2023;29:122–30.

51. Fowler JA, Viskovich S, Buckley L, et al. A call for ACTion: A systematic review of empirical evidence for the use of Acceptance and Commitment Therapy (ACT) with LGBTQI+ individuals. J Context Behav Sci 2022;25:78–89.

52. Arnold T, Haubrick KK, Klasko-Foster LB, et al. Acceptance and Commitment Therapy informed behavioral health interventions delivered by non-mental health professionals: A systematic review. J Context Behav Sci 2022;24:185–96.

53. Arch JJ, Fishbein JN, Finkelstein LB, et al. Acceptance and commitment therapy processes and mediation: Challenges and how to address them. Behav Ther 2023;54(6):971–88.

54. Onnink CM, Konstantinidou Y, Moskovich AA, et al. Acceptance and commitment therapy (ACT) for eating disorders: A systematic review of intervention studies and call to action. J Context Behav Sci 2022;26:11–28.

55. Benfer N, Spitzer EG, Bardeen JR. Efficacy of third wave cognitive behavioral therapies in the treatment of posttraumatic stress: A meta-analytic study. J Anxiety Disord 2021;78:102360.

56. Ruan J, Chen S, Liang J, et al. Acceptance and commitment therapy for insomnia and sleep quality: A systematic review and meta-analysis. J Context Behav Sci 2022;26:139–55.

57. Reardon KW, Lawrence E, Mazurek C. Adapting acceptance and commitment therapy to target intimate partner violence. Partn Abuse 2020;11(4):447–65.
58. Byrne G, O'Mahony T. Acceptance and commitment therapy (ACT) for adults with intellectual disabilities and/or autism spectrum conditions (ASC): A systematic review. J Context Behav Sci 2020;18:247–55.
59. Hayes SC, Ciarrochi J, Hofmann SG, et al. Evolving an idionomic approach to processes of change: Towards a unified personalized science of human improvement. Behav Res Ther 2022;156:104155.

Improving Exposure Therapy
Rationale and Design of an International Consortium

Jasper A.J. Smits, PhD[a],*, Jonathan S. Abramowitz, PhD[b],
Joanna J. Arch, PhD[c], Santiago Papini, PhD[d],
Rebecca A. Anderson, PhD[e], Laura J. Dixon, PhD[f],
Bronwyn M. Graham, PhD[g], Stefan G. Hofmann, PhD[h],
Jürgen Hoyer, PhD[i], Jonathan D. Huppert, PhD[j],
Jolene Jacquart, PhD[k], David Johnson, BS[l], Peter M. McEvoy, PhD[m],
Dean McKay, PhD[n], Jill Newby, PhD[o], Michael W. Otto, PhD[p],
Andre Pittig, PhD[q], Winfried Rief, PhD[r], David Rosenfield, PhD[s],
Kiara R. Timpano, PhD[t], Andre Wannemüller, PhD[u], for the
Exposure Therapy Consortium

KEYWORDS

- Exposure therapy • Treatment • Mechanism of action • Moderators • Team science
- Implementation

Continued

[a] Department of Psychology, The University of Texas at Austin, 1 University Station, Mail Code A8000, Austin, TX 78712, USA; [b] Department of Psychology, The University of North Carolina at Chapel Hill, Campus Box 3270, Chapel Hill, NC 27599, USA; [c] Department of Psychology and Neuroscience, University of Colorado Boulder, Boulder, CO, USA; [d] Department of Psychology, University of Hawai'i at Mānoa, 2530 Dole Street, Sakamaki C400, Honolulu, HI 96822, USA; [e] School of Population Health and enAble Institute, Curtin University, Bentley, Western Australia, 6102 Australia; [f] Department of Psychology, University of Mississippi, P.O. Box 1848, University, MS 38677, USA; [g] School of Psychology, UNSW Sydney, New South Wales 2052 Australia; [h] Department of Psychology, University of Marburg, Marburg 35032, Germany; [i] Technische Universität Dresden, Germany; [j] Department of Psychology, The Hebrew University of Jerusalem, Mt. Scopus, Jerusalem, 91905 Israel; [k] Department of Psychology, The University of Arizona, 1503 E. University Boulevard, Tucson, AZ 85721, USA; [l] Department of Psychological & Brain Sciences, Texas A&M University, 4235 TAMU, College Station, TX 77843, USA; [m] Centre for Clinical Interventions, Perth, Western Australia 6000, Australia; [n] Department of Psychology, Fordham University, 441 East Fordham Road, Bronx, NY 10458-5198, USA; [o] School of Psychology, UNSW Sydney at the Black Dog Institute, Hospital Road, Randwick, New South Wales 2031, Australia; [p] Department of Psychological and Brain Sciences, Boston University, 64 Cummington Mall, Boston, MA 02215, USA; [q] Translational Psychotherapy, Institute of Psychology, University of Goettingen, Germany; [r] Department of Psychology, University of Marburg, 35032 Marburg, Germany; [s] Department of Psychology, Southern Methodist University, 6425 Boaz Lane, Dallas TX 75205, USA; [t] Department of Psychology, The University of Miami, 5665 Ponce de Leon Boulevard, Coral Gables, FL 33146, USA; [u] Mental Health Research and Treatment Center, Ruhr University Bochum, Massenbergstr. 9-13, Bochum 44787, Germany
* Corresponding author.
E-mail address: smits@utexas.edu

Psychiatr Clin N Am 47 (2024) 433–444
https://doi.org/10.1016/j.psc.2024.02.008
0193-953X/24/© 2024 Elsevier Inc. All rights reserved.

psych.theclinics.com

Continued

KEY POINTS

- The Exposure Therapy Consortium (ETC) aims to facilitate team science devoted to questions surrounding the mechanisms, moderators, and associated procedural variables useful for efficacious clinical application of exposure therapy.
- ETC can promote targeted large-scale research collaborations across the translational research stages that have the potential to yield better data faster.
- ETC will facilitate training and implementation efforts that have the potential to increase exposure therapy uptake and effectiveness.

RATIONALE

Exposure therapy is a clinical strategy that involves confronting cues that activate the thoughts, emotions, and behavioral urges central to patients' presenting problems. Cues can be internal (eg, thoughts, sensations, feelings, images, or memories) and/or external (eg, situations, or people). By guiding patients to approach these cues and engage in response prevention (ie, without efforts to escape, avoid, or mitigate perceived danger), exposure therapy aims to facilitate learning opportunities that can promote symptom reduction and wellbeing.[1–3] A core and effective strategy in many established interventions for anxiety, trauma- and stress-related, and obsessive-compulsive and related disorders,[4] exposure therapy has also been applied in the treatment of substance use disorders,[5] eating disorders,[6] obesity,[7] and depression.[8]

Exposure therapy is derived from classic extinction learning approaches to altering the learned associations to stimuli, but the complexity of the learning process involved has been increasing as a result of research findings spanning the T0 (basic biomedical research) to T2 (clinical trials) translational research continuum.[9] For example, animal studies and animal-to-human translation efforts related to fear- and anxiety-related disorders have shown that the degree to which the learning of safety in response to feared cues stands apart from, is integrated with, or competes with a pre-existing fear memory depends on the degree to which the original fear learning is activated before safety learning and the similarity between the new and old learning contingencies.[10–12] There is also controversy about the relative contributions of associative and declarative learning processes in extinction in people, and ongoing clinical research has expanded the list of potential moderators of exposure therapy efficacy.[13] The result is the emergence of a complex matrix of factors that may influence exposure therapy success in the clinic; enhancement of patient care relies on the resolution of these questions about how best to engage the mechanisms of exposure therapy while understanding the contextual factors that moderate responses to this engagement. Systematic clinical research conducted with careful attention to the exact nature of exposure therapy cues and contexts holds the promise of aligning clinical intervention with advances in research on extinction. Conducting this research in a consortium allows for larger-scale studies by sharing study burden across multiple sites, refinement of design using team science, and replicability across laboratories. Moreover, larger-scale studies of this nature have the statistical power to consider the moderating role of individual difference factors that are often overlooked in basic research on extinction, where the focus has typically been on a homogenous group of rodents or human participants. Outcomes from T2 clinical research therefore have the potential to be backward translated to inform the questions being addressed in T0 basic research, and enhance the validity of basic research relevant to exposure therapy.

Echoing concerns about replicability in related literatures, initial initiatives to improve the rigor of research related to exposure therapy have included collaborations like the Research Network for the European Interdisciplinary Study of Fear and Extinction Learning as well as the Return of Fear (EIFEL-ROF) and their guidelines for the design and analysis of studies on human fear acquisition, extinction, and return of fear.[14] This article aims to complement such initiatives by establishing a global Exposure Therapy Consortium (ETC). By centralizing resources and expertise, the ETC aims to facilitate (1) team science devoted to questions surrounding the mechanisms, moderators, and associated procedural variables useful for efficacious application of exposure therapy, (2) targeted large-scale research collaborations across the translational research stages that have the potential to yield better data faster; and (3) training and implementation efforts that have the potential to increase exposure therapy uptake.

In this article, the authors describe the design of the ETC and provide an overview of initial activities. The authors hope that this overview encourages participation from researchers and clinicians who are interested in furthering research on and implementation of exposure therapy.

ORGANIZATIONAL STRUCTURE

ETC has adopted an organizational structure that can promote collaboration, productivity, and quality control, while ensuring inclusivity and equal opportunity to participate in ETC activities (**Fig. 1**). All members complete an application and agree to the terms of a memorandum of mnderstanding (see https://exposure.la.utexas.edu).

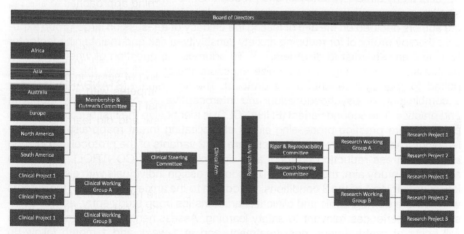

Fig. 1. ETC organizational structure. Note: The ETC has 2 organizational arms supporting its mission. Both the research and clinical arms are managed by committees. and a board of directors oversees all ETC activities. The research arm steering committee approves all research activities, supported by a rigor and reproducibility committee that is specifically tasked with providing guidance on methodology for proposed research projects. Research working groups develop and implement research projects and share data with consortium for possible follow-up (meta-) analyses. The clinical arm steering committee provides leadership to support implementation and outreach activities. It is supported by a membership and outreach committee (MOC), which is tasked with facilitating membership engagement among clinicians and clinical outreach initiatives across the globe. The MOC is supported by regional working groups to provide input and address needs particular to their region. Clinical working groups develop and facilitate training and implementation projects.

RESEARCH ACTIVITIES

The authors have established 2 research working groups to date. The first focuses on mechanisms of action. This group has reviewed extant research and (1) summarized putative mechanisms that have received empirical attention to date (eg, extinction, self-efficacy, distress tolerance, experiential avoidance, and instrumental learning) and (2) provided recommendations for future research focusing on 5 specific priority areas: conceptualization, measurement, study design/analysis, and individual/contextual differences.[13] The second working group focuses on threat extinction, a putative target for exposure therapy. This group has been piloting a standardized procedure for de novo threat conditioning studies to help ensure that variations across laboratories are not caused by the procedural differences that are evident in the conditioning literature.[14] These activities complement the publication of a book that reviews the application of exposure procedures across presenting problems.[3]

To stimulate ETC involvement and the development of new working groups and research project proposals, the authors designed a proof-of-principle study. The major aim of this pilot project is to identify and problem-solve obstacles involved in large-scale collaborative research on exposure therapy. In this next section, the authors describe this proof-of-principle project, the various obstacles they have encountered (and the solutions implemented), and the lessons learned.

Study Aims

Recognizing that coming to a design for any study may require a small rather than a large group of investigators, 4 investigators participated in a series of meetings to develop study aims, hypotheses, and procedures. Leveraging successes with 1-session large-group exposure therapy documented by Wannemüller and colleagues,[15,16] the authors decided on the aim of testing the efficacy of a 1-session large-group exposure therapy protocol for reducing anxiety sensitivity–a risk and maintaining factor for fear- and anxiety-related disorders.[17,18] To address the question of whether adding postsession processing may optimize exposure therapy efficacy, the authors proposed comparing 2 variants of the protocol. The first variant (STANDARD) includes a combination of psychoeducation and interoceptive exposure therapy modeling and practice. The second variant (ENHANCED) is identical to the first but also includes postexposure practice processing aimed at facilitating threat reappraisal (ie, safety learning). The authors proposed to compare the 2 variants of the protocol and include a general stress reduction protocol as a control condition (CONTROL). In order to achieve the study aim, the authors will randomly assign individuals with elevated anxiety sensitivity to 1 of the 3 conditions. In addition to the anxiety sensitivity, the authors will measure demographic and clinical characteristics upon study entry, as well as in-session experiences relevant to safety learning. Assessments of outcome variables will occur at pretreatment, post-treatment, and at 1-week and 1-month follow-up visits.

The preregistered hypotheses for the primary end-point are

Reduction in anxiety sensitivity from pretreatment to post-treatment will be greater in the 2 exposure conditions (combined) relative to the control condition
Reduction in anxiety sensitivity from pretreatment to post-treatment will be greater in the enhanced exposure relative to the standard exposure condition

For the secondary end-point, hypotheses are

Reduction in anxiety sensitivity from pretreatment to 1-month follow-up will be greater in the 2 exposure conditions (combined) relative to the control condition

Reduction in anxiety sensitivity from pretreatment to 1-month follow-up will be greater in the enhanced exposure relative to the standard exposure condition

Research Team

After developing the aims and procedures for the study, we approached colleagues with relevant expertise to join the investigative team. Two researchers developed a data analytical plan and power analysis for the study, agreed to oversee the randomization and analysis, and pre-registered the study (see https://clinicaltrials.gov/study/NCT05225740 and https://osf.io/uw3zs). Ten other researchers agreed to participate by collecting data at their respective sites. These researchers involved other members of their team (e.g., faculty, graduate students, research staff) to help conduct the study. Formalizing the collaboration involved reliance and data sharing agreements. We selected the University of Texas at Austin (UT) as the primary site and worked with their research office to engage the single IRB mechanism and implement necessary confidential data control plans.

Study Procedures

Critical to a quality international multisite site study involving the evaluation of a treatment protocol is removing unnecessary variability in procedures within and across sites. The authors have standardized procedures across aspects and phases of the proposed study.

Sample size determination

Power and sample size calculations were based on the ability to detect a small effect (ie, a mean difference of 0.2 standard deviation between ENHANCED and STANDARD on the primary outcome) using a cluster randomized design with a 0.1 coefficient of variation of cluster size to account for differences in recruitment across sites, an intraclass correlation of 0.02, and cluster and individual auto-correlations of 0.80 (allowing for correlations to decay across time points). With these parameters, an average group size of 20 per treatment would yield 81% power with 10 sites (ie, 200 per treatment), and 92% power with 14 sites (ie, 280 per treatment) at the .05 significance level. Note that these sample size targets provide even greater power to detect differences between the combined exposure groups and the control condition, where effect sizes are expected to be medium to large. Calculations were made using an online power and sample size calculator for cluster randomized trials.[19]

Enrollment

Because this is a nonfunded feasibility study, the authors decided to limit enrollment to university students who receive course credit for research participation. Entry criteria included ages 18 to 70, elevated anxiety sensitivity, (ie, Anxiety Sensitivity Index-3 [ASI-3][20] total score ≥23), and no history of respiratory or cardiovascular conditions, neurologic disorders, pregnancy, or other medical problems that may interfere with an ability to complete interoceptive exposure procedures. These criteria will be assessed through self-report, and eligibility will require an ASI-3 score of at least 23 on 2 administrations.[21] All sites will use existing data acquisition platforms (eg, Sona Systems, REDCap) to obtain written consent, screen, and enroll participants.

Randomization

The authors will use cluster randomization; groups of participants will be randomized to 1 of the 3 study conditions. Cluster randomization sequences (blocks of 3 stratified by site) will be computer generated such that each block of 3 sequential groups includes one of each study condition (ie, conditions do not repeat within each block).

Participants will sign up to attend a group without knowing what study condition will be randomly assigned. Study condition allocation will be concealed from the study biostatistician until analyses are completed.

Interventions
All interventions will be implemented in large-group format (targeted n ≥ 25 participants) in a classroom setting by a team of clinicians trained in exposure therapy. Aiding standardization, clinicians will deliver the interventions using a series of videos featuring one of the investigators providing instructions, education, and modeling.

Standard. The STANDARD protocol includes an orientation and psychoeducation phase (approximately 20 minutes), an exposure practice phase (approximately 75 minutes), and a task to control for the extra intervention time in the ENHANCED condition (15 minutes).

Orientation/psychoeducation phase Following general orientation, participants will watch a video that provides information about anxiety sensitivity and its role in anxiety and related disorders, as well as the rationale for interoceptive exposure practice and an overview of the intervention. Participants will then watch a video that shows a clinician and patient discussing the rationale for interoceptive exposure followed by the practice of 3 symptom induction exercises, namely spinning, straw breathing, and voluntary hyperventilation. All exercises are safe strategies to produce feared bodily sensations allowing for effective exposure therapy.[22] Following the video, participants will be asked to respond to a series of questions (with corrective feedback offered by clinicians) to help ensure that psychoeducation resulted in an understanding of the model of exposure therapy and its procedures.

Exposure practice phase Participants will rotate in smaller subgroups through 3 group-based exposure exercises (30 seconds of spinning, 1 minute of straw breathing, 1 minute of hyperventilation), each led by a team of clinicians using separate classrooms. Each exposure exercise involves 5 repeated trials interspersed with ratings of anticipated and actual perceived threat and fear.

Control task To control for the time involved in the postprocessing exercise in the ENHANCED condition, participants will complete a set of questions regarding the exercises (without a specific attempt to highlight the discrepancy between anticipated and actual outcomes). Following completion of the control task, all participants will reconvene in the main classroom for a group-based debriefing. The clinicians will be available to offer assistance with regulating the distress resulting from exposure practice should that be needed.

Enhanced. Participants assigned to ENHANCED will receive an intervention that is identical to STANDARD with the addition of a 15-minute postprocessing exercise that precedes the group-based debriefing. This exercise starts with a brief video that shows a clinician and patient discussing the learning that occurred during exposure practice. Following the video, participants will be asked to write out responses to a series of questions aimed at facilitating safety learning. Clinicians will engage the group in a brief discussion to aid processing.

Control. Participants assigned to this condition will receive the same amount in minutes of stress management training (SMT), which is designed to help people better cope with feelings of anxiety that accompany high levels of anxiety sensitivity. SMT will involve video-delivered group instruction, facilitated by clinicians, in healthy ways to experience and cope with stress whenever difficult situations arise. Participants will learn about the components of the stress response, including its positive and negative consequences. SMT will also teach participants ways to maintain a healthy lifestyle, targeting things like nutrition, exercise, and sleep hygiene.

Assessment

Data collection and entry procedures were standardized across sites. Specifically, the prescreens and follow-up surveys will be collected electronically, while data collected during the session (baseline, within-session, and postintervention measures) will be recorded via paper and pencil and entered into REDCap by research teams following the session. To ensure data entry integrity, the primary outcome measure (ASI-3) will be double coded, and all data entered from the paper and pencil measures will be checked by multiple research team members.

To facilitate standardization, the REDCap database was developed and pilot-tested at the primary site before deployment to collaborating institutions. Once the database was deemed reliable, REDCap XML files were sent to research teams so that each site would have the identical database structure. The standardized REDCap database included additional sections for Institutional Review Board (IRB) reporting, participant tracking, and postsession reporting. These supplemental sections provided ways for research teams to keep track of participation, compensation, and any potential adverse events. Once all sessions are completed by a collaborating site, de-identified REDCap data will be sent to the relying institution and stored on secure, encrypted cloud servers. All data entered manually will be checked for inaccuracies before data analysis.

Primary outcome measure

The ASI-3 is an 18-item self-report used to assess concern associated with possible negative consequences of anxiety-related symptoms. Responses are rated on a 5-point Likert scale ranging from 0 (very little) to 4 (very much) and summed to create a total score. Total scores range from 0 to 72. The authors selected this measure because of its sound psychometric properties.[20] Readers are referred to a supplement (https://osf.io/7u6ef) that describes measures included in this protocol for screening and to achieve secondary aims.

Data Analysis

The preregistered analysis plan and any subsequent modifications are publicly available on the Open Science Framework (https://osf.io/uw3zs). Following intention-to-treat principles, all participants who attend their group will be included in the analyses. All analyses will use mixed effects (multilevel) modeling to account for the nested structure of the data: repeated measures (level 1), nested within participants (level 2), nested within groups (level 3), nested within sites (level 4). The primary outcome model (ASI-3) will include fixed effects of phase (pretreatment, post-treatment, 1-week follow-up, 1-month follow-up), condition (exposure-enhanced, exposure-standard, control), and a condition-by-phase interaction. Helmert coding will be used for the conditions to make the comparisons necessary to test the hypotheses (ie, both exposure conditions versus control; exposure-enhanced versus exposure standard). The authors will also fit alternative models (eg, piecewise growth curves) and select the best-fitting model based on AIC/BIC. Primary end-point hypotheses will be tested by comparing changes in ASI-3 from pretreatment to post-treatment. Secondary end-point hypotheses will be tested by comparing changes in ASI-3 from pretreatment to 1-month-follow-up. Across all analyses, group differences will be considered significant at the standard $P<.05$ level. Each estimate will include a

95% confidence interval and a Cohen D effect size. Analyses will be conducted using the open-source statistical software *R*. After completion of the trial and publication of results, de-identified data, analysis code, and output will be posted on the OSF repository for this project (https://osf.io/h4875/).

Training

To minimize variability in study administration and implementation, the authors generated brief training modules for staff and clinicians and made these available on a study Web site (https://exposure.la.utexas.edu/research/projects/project-1/etc-training-modules). Each of these modules provides an overview of and education in procedures (eg., screening, assessment, treatment) and systems (REDCap). The training for clinicians also includes a brief video-recorded workshop. Site investigators will be responsible to ensure that staff and clinicians have completed the relevant training and are prepared to participate in the study.

Challenges

Team science brings with it a series of challenges that are interpersonal and organizational in nature and reflect the complexities inherent in having highly productive people from disparate institutions agree on common research methods that may nonetheless intersect with institution-specific barriers to completion. Fortunately, guidance is available for anticipating and addressing some of these challenges.[23] Significant challenges can also arise from outside the collaborative network. For example, after multiple delays caused by the COVID-19 (coronavirus disease 2019) pandemic, the authors have observed several challenges implementing the study as planned. First, obtaining IRB approval has required high levels of organization and communication from all sites. In some instances, slower communication between review boards or with lawyers about data sharing has resulted in minor delays in startups at collaborating sites. Using the single IRB mechanism where possible aids efficiency; yet, the burden and responsibilities of managing documentation for multiple sites befalls the primary institution. Second, the decision to require REDCap presented challenges for some sites. Institutions that do not have a REDCap license must access REDCap at the primary site, which requires formal appointments at this site and the necessary training for new users of the REDCap system. The materials that the authors have posted on the study training Web site and providing opportunities to consult with primary site researchers have helped remedy this obstacle. Third, this study involves sites across different continents and thus requires translation of study materials. To date, all study materials are available in English, German, Arabic, and Hebrew; yet this required considerable effort, including extra piloting of the protocols to ensure the translations were understood as intended. At the same time, the ubiquitousness of English (eg, in movies and shows) made subtitling the English videos quite feasible.

Perhaps because of the COVID-19 pandemic, the authors also observed changes in student participation in research studies. Specifically, across sites, enrollment rates for in-person studies have decreased relative to before the pandemic. Credit points toward study course requirements may also be insufficient to motivate large numbers of university students to participate in exposure groups, compared with clients presenting to mental health clinics because of distress and disability resulting from their anxiety sensitivity and associated panic symptoms. Thus, although university students were targeted because of their accessibility, it has been more difficult than anticipated to engage them in group therapy sessions. This can result in substantial delays and rescheduling of sessions, resulting in additional administrative burden for research coordinators and posing continuity issues when students involved in facilitating projects are required to meet deadlines for thesis submissions and graduations. As a result, the authors have made the following changes to the protocol.

First, although keeping 25 as the minimum target group size, all sites will run all scheduled sessions regardless of group size.

Second, depending on the group size, sites can either rotate subgroups of participants through the 3 exposure tasks or complete all three with the full group. For the former option, sites can form 3 exposure practice stations in separate classrooms and assign clinicians to run these for 3 subgroups. Sites are instructed to use the same approach across the STANDARD and ENHANCED conditions at their site.

Third, to maintain a reasonable clinician to participant ratio, sites can employ as many as 2 clinicians per exposure practice station to as few as 1 clinician for smaller groups.

Fourth, because of the unexpected reduced participant flow, sites have the option to complete data collection (running 3 groups) across multiple semesters. Secondary analyses may be designed to test whether treatment delivery parameters (eg, group size, use of subgroups, number of clinicians, and date of the session) predict treatment outcome or moderate the between-group effects.

CLINICAL ACTIVITIES

The authors have established 1 clinical working group to date focused on creating a resource repository to support clinician training and delivery of exposure therapy for a wide range of presenting concerns. The Evidence-Based Practice Resource Repository (https://exposure.la.utexas.edu/clinical/resources) is a database of peer-reviewed research articles, empirically supported clinical guides and treatment manuals, and educational videos and tools that allows clinicians to easily locate useful information and tools to aid the delivery of effective exposure therapy. In addition, this working group has developed several worksheets (eg, exposure lists, monitoring distress during exposures, and tracking out-of-session exposure practice) and made these available in multiple languages.

BENEFITS OF ENGAGEMENT IN THE EXPOSURE THERAPY CONSORTIUM

ETC was organized to provide benefit to the field by facilitating larger-scale studies that can be conducted with lower burden across multiple collaborating sites (with lower sample size demand at each of the participating sites). This strategy has the additional benefit of engaging multiple minds in the design and honing of proposed projects and affords automatic replication across sites using a standardized protocol. In addition to the enhanced research productivity and potentially higher impact of papers associated with team science collaborations,[24] investigators in ETC can reap the benefits of being exposed to

A broader set of research measures, methods, and technical skills within one's area of study

The unique issues and proposed solutions faced by researchers at each site

The automatic assumptions and well-thought theoretic conceptualizations held by multiple researchers within a subfield

The potential to by-pass early stage funding needs as projects and protocols are developed, tested, and replicated across sites

The opportunity to conduct larger sample size studies on detailed questions that may not be ready for large-scale funding requests

International leaders to build local capacity for clinicians (eg, clinical skills), re-searchers (eg, trial methodology and coordination), and students

Potential for competitiveness for research funding locally, nationally, and internationally

CONCLUSIONS AND FUTURE DIRECTIONS

In conclusion, ETC has successfully implemented an organizational structure aimed at fostering collaboration, productivity, and quality control. The establishment of research working groups targeting specific areas such as mechanisms of action and fear extinction signifies an organized and focused approach to tackling complex issues in exposure therapy. These groups have not only developed research agendas but have also contributed to the academic community through peer-reviewed articles and books. A proof-of-principle study has been initiated to further encourage collab-orative research by identifying and resolving challenges related to large scale projects. Additionally, a clinical working group has been set up to bolster clinician training and practice, featuring an extensive evidence-based practice resource repository and a range of useful clinical tools available in multiple languages.

Despite the strides that have been made, challenges remain. ETC has made use of technology to facilitate global collaboration while adopting a pragmatic approach of initiating projects within smaller, more localized groups. This strategy has proven effective in addressing logistical issues while maintaining the momentum of the con-sortium's various activities. Overall, ETC has laid a robust foundation for advancing exposure therapy research and clinical practice through collaborative efforts, thereby making significant contributions to the field. Relatedly, although restrictions on in-person research have eased, difficulties in recruiting participants are ongoing and likely to persist. Although challenging, these difficulties also present opportunities for innovation.

Looking to the future, the ETC could focus on expanding its working groups to cover more specialized areas within exposure therapy, potentially leading to additional multi-site trials for robust and generalizable findings. Technology integration, such as devel-oping a dedicated platform for asynchronous collaboration, could alleviate the challenges of coordinating across time zones. The ETC is also well positioned to develop and test the feasibility of digital delivery of exposure therapy, which could enhance participant recruitment rates and aid in the democratization of access to exposure therapy globally. Another key area could be forming a world-wide conference on exposure therapy, international partnerships, and localized hubs to facilitate easier collaboration and to expand the consortium's reach. This international focus could also extend to offering specialized training to clinicians worldwide, localizing clinical re-sources into additional languages, and engaging in policy advocacy to standardize exposure therapy protocols globally. Further, the consortium could capitalize on its data accumulation by employing advanced analytics for deeper insights and predictive modeling. Public awareness campaigns could be another avenue to combat negative beliefs associated with exposure therapy (and stigma of psychotherapy more broadly) and to disseminate evidence-based information. By pursuing these directions, the ETC has the potential to not only deepen its existing research but also expand its impact in advancing the science and practice of exposure therapy on a global scale.

DISCLOSURE

Funding Support: Author effort was supported as follows: Dr J.A.J. Smits (NIMH R01MH125951), Dr S.G. Hofmann (Alexander von Humboldt Foundation, Germany and Hessische Ministerium für Wissenschaft und Kunst), Dr J. Newby (NHMRC 2008839), Australia, and Dr M.W. Otto (NIMH R01 MH125949), United States. These funding sources had no role in the content or the decision to publish this article.Dr J.A.J. Smits receives funding from National Institute on Drug Abuse (NIDA R01DA047933), United States, the National Cancer Institute (NCI R01CA273221), United States, and Department of Defense (TP220002), United States, and compensation and royalties from various publishers. Dr J.J. Arch receives current research funding from the National Institutes of Health, United States/National Institute of Nursing Research (R01NR018479). Dr S G. Hofmann receives financial support by the Alexander von Humboldt Foundation (as part of the Alexander von Humboldt Professur) and the Hessische Ministerium für Wissenschaft und Kunst (as part of the LOEWE Spitzenprofessur). He also receives compensation for his work as editor from SpringerNature and royalties and payments for his work from various publishers. Dr P.M. McEvoy receives compensation from The Guilford Press, Elsevier, Cambridge University Press, and McGraw-Hill Education. Dr J. Newby receives funding from the Australian National Medical Research Council, and the Medical Research Future Fund. Dr M.W. Otto receives compensation as an advisor to Big Health and receives grant support from National Institute of Mental Health, United States, NIDA, and Big Health. Dr D. Rosenfield reports funding from NIMH, NCI, National Center for Complementary and Integrative Health, United States, and the Patient-Centered Outcomes Research Institute, United States. He also receives compensation from several scientific journals and from Rosenfield Analytics. Dr W.Rief received honoraria from Boehringer Ingelheim for talks on Post Covid, and he receives royalties from book publications from different publishers. All other authors report no conflicts of interest.

REFERENCES

1. Abramowitz JS, Deacon BJ, Whiteside SPH. Exposure therapy for anxiety: principles and practice. New York, NY, USA: Guilford Publications; 2019.
2. Smits JAJ, Powers MB, Otto MW. Personalized exposure therapy: a person-centered transdiagnostic approach. New York, NY, USA: Oxford University Press; 2019.
3. Smits JAJ, Jacquart J, Abramowitz J, et al, editors. Clinical guide to exposure therapy: beyond phobias. Springer International Publishing; 2022. https://doi.org/10.1007/978-3-031-04927-9.
4. Carpenter JK, Andrews LA, Witcraft SM, et al. Cognitive behavioral therapy for anxiety and related disorders: a meta-analysis of randomized placebo-controlled trials. Depress Anxiety 2018;35(6):502–14.
5. McHugh RK, Kosiba JD, Chase AR. Exposure therapy in the treatment of substance use disorders. In: Smits JAJ, Jacquart J, Abramowitz J, et al, editors. Clinical guide to exposure therapy: beyond phobias. New York, NY, USA: Springer International Publishing; 2022. p. 261–76. https://doi.org/10.1007/978-3-031-04927-9_14.
6. Becker CB, Farrell NR, Waller G. Using exposure therapy for eating disorders. In: Smits JAJ, Jacquart J, Abramowitz J, et al, editors. Clinical guide to exposure therapy: beyond phobias. New York, NY, USA: Springer International Publishing; 2022. p. 277–97. https://doi.org/10.1007/978-3-031-04927-9_15.
7. Boutelle KN, Eichen DM, Virzi NE. Exposure exercises for overeating, binge eating, and obesity. In: Smits JAJ, Jacquart J, Abramowitz J, et al, editors. Clinical guide to exposure therapy: beyond phobias. New York, NY, USA: Springer

International Publishing; 2022. p. 299–316. https://doi.org/10.1007/978-3-031-04927-9_16.

8. Hayes AM, Yasinski C, Alpert E. The application of exposure principles to the treatment of depression. In: Smits JAJ, Jacquart J, Abramowitz J, et al, editors. Clinical guide to exposure therapy: beyond phobias. New York, NY, USA: Springer International Publishing; 2022. p. 317–45. https://doi.org/10.1007/978-3-031-04927-9_17.

9. Richter J, Pittig A, Hollandt M, et al. Bridging the gaps between basic science and cognitive-behavioral treatments for anxiety disorders in routine care: Current status and future demands. Z Psychol 2017;225(3):252–67.

10. Gershman SJ, Monfils MH, Norman KA, et al. In: The computational nature of memory modification6. Elife; 2017. p. e23763. https://doi.org/10.7554/eLife.23763.

11. Kredlow MA, Eichenbaum H, Otto MW. Memory creation and modification: Enhancing the treatment of psychological disorders. Am Psychol 2018;73(3):269–85.

12. Raskin M, Monfils MH. Reconsolidation and fear extinction: an update. Curr Top Behav Neurosci 2023. https://doi.org/10.1007/7854_2023_438.

13. Benito K, Pittig A, Abramowitz J, et al. Mechanisms of change in exposure therapy for anxiety and related disorders: a research agenda. Clinical Psychological Science. 2023. in press.

14. Lonsdorf TB, Menz MM, Andreatta M, et al. Don't fear "fear conditioning": methodological considerations for the design and analysis of studies on human fear acquisition, extinction, and return of fear. Neurosci Biobehav Rev 2017;77:247–85.

15. Wannemueller A, Fasbender A, Kampmann Z, et al. Large-group one-session treatment: a feasibility study of exposure combined with applied tension or diaphragmatic breathing in highly blood-injury-injection fearful individuals. Front Psychol 2018;9:1534.

16. Wannemueller A, Schaumburg S, Tavenrath S, et al. Large-group one-session treatment: Feasibility and efficacy in 138 individuals with phobic fear of flying. Behav Res Ther 2020;135:103735.

17. Otto MW, Eastman A, Lo S, et al. Anxiety sensitivity and working memory capacity: Risk factors and targets for health behavior promotion. Clin Psychol Rev 2016;49:67–78.

18. Smits JAJ, Otto MW, Powers MB, et al. Anxiety sensitivity as a transdiagnostic treatment target. In: Smits JAJ, Otto MW, Powers MB, et al, editors. The clinician's guide to anxiety sensitivity treatment and assessment. 1st edition. San Diego, CA: Academic Press; 2018. p. 1–5.

19. Hemming K, Kasza J, Hooper R, et al. A tutorial on sample size calculation for multiple-period cluster randomized parallel, cross-over and stepped-wedge trials using the Shiny CRT Calculator. Int J Epidemiol 2020;49(3):979–95.

20. Taylor S, Zvolensky MJ, Cox BJ, et al. Robust dimensions of anxiety sensitivity: development and initial validation of the Anxiety Sensitivity Index-3. Psychol Assess 2007;19(2):176–88.

21. Marsic A, Broman-Fulks JJ, Berman ME. The effects of measurement frequency and timing on anxiety sensitivity scores. Cogn Ther Res 2010;35(5):463–8.

22. Antony MM, Ledley DR, Liss A, et al. Responses to symptom induction exercises in panic disorder. Behav Res Ther 2006;44(1):85–98.

23. Bennett LM, Gadlin H. Collaboration and team science: from theory to practice. J Investig Med 2012;60(5):768–75.

24. Wuchty S, Jones BF, Uzzi B. The increasing dominance of teams in production of knowledge. Science 2007;316(5827):1036–9.

Moving?

Make sure your subscription moves with you!

To notify us of your new address, find your **Clinics Account Number** (located on your mailing label above your name), and contact customer service at:

Email: journalscustomerservice-usa@elsevier.com

800-654-2452 (subscribers in the U.S. & Canada)
314-447-8871 (subscribers outside of the U.S. & Canada)

Fax number: 314-447-8029

Elsevier Health Sciences Division
Subscription Customer Service
3251 Riverport Lane
Maryland Heights, MO 63043

*To ensure uninterrupted delivery of your subscription, please notify us at least 4 weeks in advance of move.

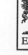

Printed and bound by CPI Group (UK) Ltd, Croydon, CR0 4YY

03/10/2024

01040468-0017